Too Tired To Think

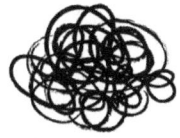

A practical guide to living
with long-term fatigue

Chronic Fatigue Syndrome (ME/CFS)
Long-COVID
Fibromyalgia

Sarah Vizer

Published by:
Sarah Vizer, Queensland, Australia.
sarahvizer.com/tootiredtothink

Copyright © 2024 Sarah Vizer. All rights reserved.

No part of this book may be reproduced, stored in any retrieval system, or transmitted in any form or by any means, electronic, mechanical, photocopying, recording or otherwise, without the prior written permission of the copyright holder, except for the use of brief quotations in a book review.

For permission requests, contact Sarah Vizer: sarah@sarahvizer.com

The information contained in this book is for educational purposes only. It is the result of the research and experience of the author. While the information offered is believed to be true and accurate at the time of publication, the author does not accept any legal responsibility for errors or omissions that may have been made.

This book is not intended to provide a medical or mental health diagnosis or substitute for medical or mental health advice. The author is not, and does not hold themselves to be, a doctor, physician or any other medical professional (Medical Provider). The author is not, and does not hold themselves to be, a psychologist, psychiatrist, psychotherapist, counsellor, or social worker (Mental Health Provider).

You must take complete responsibility for your own physical health and emotional wellbeing. You are advised to always consult a qualified medical practitioner and seek your own individualised medical and mental health care.

All characters in this book are based on real, commonly reported experiences, but the characters are fictitious. Any resemblance to persons is purely coincidental and unintended.

ISBN: 978-1-7636929-0-9
E-book ISBN: 978-1-7636929-1-6

For Demian, Oliver and Savannah
who provide me with the oxygen
of their unconditional love and support.

"I am not what happened to me.
I am what I choose to become."

– Carl Jung

Table of Contents

Preface - The Reality of Our Times *1*

Introduction **5**
    Chapter 1 - A Framework for Recovery 14

Physical Reality…Nurturing a Tired Body **27**
    Chapter 2 - Different Origins, Similar Challenges 30
    Chapter 3 - The Impact of Post-Exertional Malaise 45
    Chapter 4 - Managing Finite Energy 55
    Chapter 5 - Learning to Love Pacing 73
        Physical Summary *82*

Emotional Reality…Riding the Rollercoaster **83**
    Chapter 6 - A Rollercoaster of Emotions 88
    Chapter 7 - Unhelpful Thought Patterns 99
    Chapter 8 - Developing a Healing Mindset 108
    Chapter 9 - Preparing for Those Dark Days 129
    Chapter 10 - Managing the People in Your Life 138
        Emotional Summary *151*

Medical Reality…Navigating Cracked Systems **153**
    Chapter 11 - Utilising a Team of Practitioners 158

Chapter 12 - Hurdles Within Medical Systems 171
Chapter 13 - Taking Control of your Medical Reality 180
   Medical Summary...193

Getting the Help you Need…What Works and What Doesn't...... 194
Chapter 14 - Lifestyle, Back to Basics...197
Chapter 15 - Becoming a Pacing Expert...215
Chapter 16 - Moving with Care, Not Out of Obligation 227
Chapter 17 - Building Your Supportive Team..233
Chapter 18 - Navigating Work Situations 242
Chapter 19 - Ways of Feeling Mindful 252
Chapter 20 - Restoring Energy and Cultivating Joy...............................258
Chapter 21 - Maintaining Perspective 265

New Reality — A Message of Hope.. 275

Acknowledgments..280
Glossary 283
About the author 291

Preface

The Reality of Our Times

'Breaking news…the global health emergency is over,' reports the World Health Organization in May 2023. Except it's not for those still feeling the effects of the COVID-19 post-viral condition commonly known as long-COVID. These are the unseen stories that make up our current uncharted epidemic. Up to 65 million people globally[1] are suffering with long-COVID, with one of the most common symptoms being long-term fatigue.

Add to this the estimated 17-24 million[2] already suffering from myalgic encephalomyelitis/chronic fatigue syndrome (ME/CFS) and the potential 2-4% of the population[3] living with fibromyalgia, and you start to see how staggering the global numbers of long-term fatigue really are.

---

1   Statistics from January 2023, based on a conservative estimated incidence of 10% of infected people developing long-COVID from the more than 651 million documented COVID-19 cases worldwide. Cases are still increasing daily. Article link — www.nature.com/articles/s41579-022-00846-2
2   Statistics from CDC estimates. Emerge Australia reports that studies estimate 0.4 to 1% of the population have ME/CFS. These are estimates only, and perhaps the true extent of ME/CFS is unknown.
3   Statistics widely vary, but a 2018 paper by Winfried Hauser MD and Mary-Ann Fitzcharles MD referenced by the National Library of Medicine finds that fibromyalgia occurs in all populations throughout the world, with a prevalence of between 2 to 4% in general populations.

Long-term fatigue is defined as extreme fatigue lasting longer than six months, with symptoms that worsen through physical or mental activity and that are not relieved by rest or sleep[4]. It is not discriminatory in who it affects, leaving no nation untouched and includes all ages, genders and backgrounds. Up to 80% of ME/CFS cases are women, with 25% so affected they are effectively house-bound, sometimes even confined to their bed[5]. This trend is even further pronounced in fibromyalgia, which affects women 10 to 20 times more than men[6].

These are the statistics, but what they don't reveal are the devastating effects that living with long-term fatigue entails.

Tiredness, even fatigue, is a common experience that most of us can relate to, but long-term fatigue is different. It's a misleading, even polite-sounding term that disrespects the utter exhaustion present in every cell of the body. It's usually accompanied by a whole raft of other debilitating symptoms that contribute to a gruelling journey, which can persist for months, even years.

Fatigue goes far beyond the physical symptoms, affecting mental and emotional wellbeing as well. It replaces vibrancy and aspirations with limitation and trade-offs. Living in societies that value contribution, this frequently leads to feelings of isolation, frustration and despair.

Fatigue often hits people in their prime, as it did this author, overwhelming the lives of those it touches. It impacts their ability to work and care for their families, their relationships and their overall quality of life. In some cases, it can even be life-threatening, increasing the risk of accidents and other health problems.

---

4 Based on the definition and criteria for diagnosing ME/CFS. Long-term fatigue as a term covers the conditions of ME/CFS, fibromyalgia and long-COVID. These can all have ME/CFS in common within the diagnosis.
5 Statistics from Emerge Australia - www.emerge.org.au/what-is-me-cfs
6 Statistics based on the work of Dr David Brady, author of 'The Fibro Fix'.

Our medical communities need help diagnosing and treating this condition. How can there *still* not be consensus that fatigue is even a condition, let alone the lack of a common method of treatment for doctors to follow? Fatigue patients are frequently misdiagnosed, and treatment becomes hit or miss — usually focused on the management of symptoms[7].

You can see for yourself the effects of serious physical illnesses like a stroke or cancer. People flock around, deliver meals, ask what they can do to help, offer their support for as long as it is needed.

In contrast, ME/CFS, fibromyalgia and long-COVID are often hidden conditions, suffering the same fate as many of the over 1 billion people globally living with a non-visible disability[8]. Those affected seem deceptively healthy on the outside and as a result experience a whole gamut of physical, mental and emotional turmoil.

Others might offer to help for a while, but those offers tend to fade over time. It is no surprise that we hear reports of people experiencing unbidden thoughts where they might fleetingly wish for a more tangible illness instead, even cancer in extreme cases, just to have something 'fixable' to receive the support they need.

Without better diagnosis and treatment, these are the lengths people may be driven to when experiencing long-term fatigue.

There is some light at the end of the tunnel. The COVID-19 pandemic has highlighted the issue of long-term fatigue in a way that has not been seen before. Long-COVID research is leading to better understanding and more treatment options for the ME/CFS community. As a result, this community

---

7 The US Centers for Disease Control and Prevention (CDC) outright states there is no cure or approved treatment for ME/CFS, rather it becomes around the management of symptoms. You can find out more about the CDC's advice for ME/CFS at: www.cdc.gov/me-cfs
8 Statistics and a list of hidden disabilities are available from Hidden Disabilities Sunflower. Access the site here — hiddendisabilitiesstore.com

now holds more hope for better care, better science and more standardised and advanced treatments to come.

This book explores the reality of living with long-term fatigue, based on lived experiences. It examines methods of managing the physical challenges, navigating the emotional rollercoaster, advocating for yourself, finding the right support, implementing helpful practices and educating those around you. By the end, you will have a solid understanding of the challenges and opportunities that lie ahead.

This is the reality of our times: the quest to feel seen and heard while navigating the physical, emotional and medical realities of long-term fatigue — the hidden struggles silently affecting the lives of millions of people around the world.

Introduction

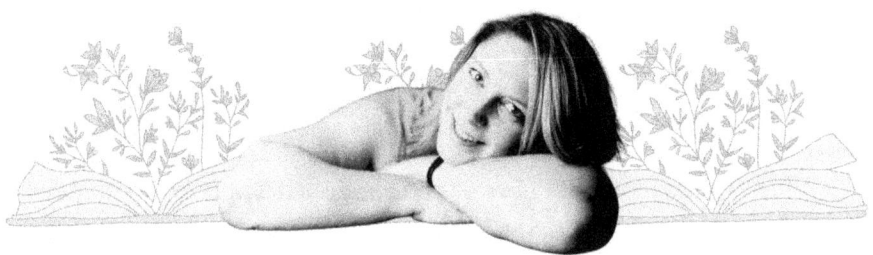

Hi, I'm Sarah Vizer. I'm a vibrant, motivated type of person. I'm also someone who has lived with the devastating effects of long-term fatigue for more than seven years.

It was July 2017 when I took a two-week break from my job as a corporate consultant for one of the Big Four in Australia. Despite being desperate to return to the workplace, I was never able to do so. I later discovered I was suffering from the effects of what had started out as corporate burnout and later developed into myalgic encephalomyelitis/chronic fatigue syndrome (ME/CFS). I recognise the official term for this condition is ME/CFS, but I was first introduced to it as chronic fatigue syndrome and will use this term throughout the book when referring to my own fatigue condition experience[9].

---

9   The official term is ME/CFS. The community has long fought for this term to be officially recognised as it represents the seriousness of a genuine medical condition. I was first told I had chronic fatigue syndrome and continue to use that term. I find it to be less clinical, and helps people better understand what my condition entails. For these reasons, ME/CFS will be referred to as 'chronic fatigue syndrome' when referencing my fatigue condition as I experience it.

During this time, chronic fatigue syndrome ruled my life in so many ways. I felt the lows and the even deeper lows that accompany this condition. I discovered firsthand what it's like to live at the extremes:

- When your energy is so low it becomes a choice between feeding yourself or having a shower
- When you desperately want to attend a long-anticipated event with family and friends, but your body won't allow it and an aching loneliness seeps in
- When it feels like every fibre of your body aches and even lying down feels too hard. Forget thinking. This book was almost called *Too Tired to Rest*!

I also knew what it was like to experience it on an everyday basis:

- When you wake up unrefreshed, but push on because you desperately don't want to let anyone down
- When you cry secret tears of exhaustion because you're sick of trying to explain your tears to others
- When you have a great day and accidently overdo it, only to pay the exhausting price for days afterwards

Needless to say, there were some dark times across those seven years. But it's not all bad. There were plenty of good times and even some great achievements in there as well. I've recently felt the joyous highs that arise from feeling energetically alive again and like life is somewhat back on track, albeit a different track from what I first imagined.

Too Tired to Think is *not* a sad story. Rather it's a book about hope. You'll read about my journey — one that has been triumphant in the outcome — but I am also honest about the frustration and hurt it has taken.

I'm continuing to morph my life along a new trajectory, adapting to the fatigue that still inhabits my body. I can see the benefits that living with fatigue has brought to my life. I've had a major rethink about what I want for my future. I've changed my goals and started shooting for new and different heights. I've sought advice and opened my mind to new ways — things like meditation, pacing myself, career changes, even expanding my friendship circle. I've read countless books, listened to podcasts, discovered ideas that inspire me. I've tapped into what we call 'purpose' and 'passion', and allowed that to lead me forward.

Most of all, I'm happy!

When you're in the messy middle of your long-term fatigue struggle, seeing all of this is often not possible. It's only now I'm emerging from its tenacious grip and finding my new normal that I can truly recognise the growth it has brought.

One thing has become very clear from this time — what I've experienced has been a course-correction and a gift. Burnout was the trigger of my chronic fatigue syndrome and this came out of living a life that wasn't right for me. And I wasn't doing anything about it. So, when my mind wouldn't listen, my body shut down, effectively making the course-correcting decision on my behalf. Calling chronic fatigue syndrome a gift might seem like a bit of a stretch, but it has allowed me to grow, changing the trajectory of my future.

Anyone can get sick. Enduring the battle with a condition that leads to long-term fatigue reveals the depth and strength of a person. By continuing to fight even when you feel at your weakest demonstrates your admirable resilience. From there, it's how you rebuild, putting yourself back together, that makes you the person you will become.

It can be magic and hell all rolled into one!

You're here because you have someone in your life who has been affected by fatigue — either yourself directly or a parent, partner, patient, friend, co-worker, neighbour or other loved one. This book is about what it takes to truly navigate a chronic, hidden condition such as fatigue over the long term.

If you in any way, shape or form are going through a debilitating condition that leads to long-term fatigue, it will guide you to find the support and understanding that you so sorely need and deserve. It will also assist your loved ones and medical professional team towards better understanding.

Those who live around and care for people with long-term fatigue will find value understanding how better to support them, strengthening your bonds and allowing your relationship to flourish based on mutual understanding.

Healthcare practitioners can use this book to understand the patient experience and as a tool to recommend to their patients. This will support your own recommendations and help each client understand their condition more holistically than they might otherwise.

It has also proven relevant for people with other conditions leading to fatigue, or indeed those with no identifiable medical fatigue condition who are still facing the reality of long-term fatigue.

As a researcher of both facts and stories, my goal is to bring to life both the journey and solutions from those of us who are navigating this difficult condition to help all of us in a meaningful way. I am not a medical professional; rather I am someone who has gone through a rough period, and wants to share my training and experience. This has allowed me to write this book in a way that is sensitive to the challenges experienced when navigating long-term fatigue.

The following outlines ways that you, the reader, can get the most out of this book.

How you can use this book (especially when you're tired!)

Too Tired to Think **is a general guide, summarising the common challenges of long-term fatigue.** I encourage you to lift yourself out of the detail when reading it.

While it covers the big picture across the conditions of ME/CFS, fibromyalgia and long-COVID and the common long-term fatigue challenges people with these conditions face, you will not find an exhaustive list of symptoms or specific treatments as these seem to be constantly evolving.

Instead, the focus is on what doesn't change…the foundations for getting the help you need to manage these conditions.

You have a choice in how you read this book. What I've set out to achieve is a structure of easily digestible chapters that you can pick up and put down, knowing this is required for so many of us with long-term fatigue.

If you're feeling okay, then feel free to start at the beginning and work your way through the book chapter by chapter.

If you're currently feeling the effects of fatigue, reading a book cover-to-cover might be beyond you. In this case start with Chapter 1, reading a few pages at a time. It might be you step in and out of the bits you need right now, and you will most likely find different areas to revisit as you further reflect on your experiences. After Chapter 1, you might want to jump straight into the help and guidance section, then come back to the earlier chapters once your energy improves.

Here's a summary of what you can expect from each section:

Framework for recovery — Chapter 1 provides you with a model for your marathon journey to improvement and 'recovery'. This is often not recovery in the truest sense of the word, rather discovering a new normal way of life.

Physical reality — Chapters 2 to 5 are about getting a handle on what is happening to you right now. This section covers your symptoms, the impact of activity (particularly when you overdo it), how to manage finite energy and an introduction to pacing — arguably *the* best strategy available for managing your fatigue.

Emotional reality — Chapters 6 to 10 are around navigating the highs and lows of this condition. You may not be ready for this section just yet and that's okay, but you may also be very ready to delve into creating an easier frame of mind. This section looks at the rollercoaster of emotions you may be feeling, your mindset and how to identify unhelpful thought patterns, developing a healing mindset, preparing for darker days and how to manage the people in your life.

> A bonus downloadable e-book providing relationship support and conversation starters to spark those valuable discussions with those around you is also available.
> You can get your copy at: www.sarahvizer.com/tootiredtothink

Medical reality — Chapters 11 to 13 help you navigate the difficult world of medical options and practitioners, with the aim of getting the care you need. This section looks at advocating for yourself, putting together an effective multidisciplinary team of professionals, finding your 'gems' and dealing with the various hurdles experienced by those who have gone before you.

Getting the help you need — Chapters 14 to 21 are the practical application of the earlier information, building the foundation of good practice to manage your condition. You can jump straight to this section if you have very little energy right now and just want some quick actions to implement straight away.

If there is a particular topic that you're currently struggling with then head straight to that section. This book is about your own personal journey, so just start somewhere!

At the end, you will also find a glossary of common fatigue-related terms that you may not be familiar with yet. It will be useful for getting a quick definition if and when you feel lost about what something means.

We can relate to the experiences of each other. At the start of each chapter, you will find short vignettes or stories of others who are experiencing long-term fatigue.

Stories elevate the content from secondhand knowledge to tangible lived experiences. These are the experiences of those navigating long-term fatigue across all walks of life. They are important as they represent an increasing number of people who struggle with long-term fatigue. The more I research, the more I realise the magnitude of the problem, particularly now we have so many people around the world affected by long-COVID.

I have protected the identity of the people involved by creating characters rather than using real people, including names, ages, professions and geographical locations. Fictional though they are, they highlight consistent themes and illustrate the challenges and frustrations commonly faced within the conditions of ME/CFS, fibromyalgia and long-COVID.

I have used my own accumulated experience along with collecting the experiences of hundreds (if not thousands) of others. Supplementing the verbal interviews, gaining insights from social media groups and community forums has been a breakthrough. It has felt like I've found 'my people' who intimately understood these conditions firsthand and are not afraid to share the good, the bad and the ugly of their experiences. I am incredibly grateful for the candour and courage shown in these interviews, groups and forums as people pull back the curtain on reality.

Reading their stories showed me the commonalities with my own experiences, but also the vast variations. No one post is a source of truth for all, but consistent themes emerge from multiple sources that together form a picture, guideposts for how 'typical' experiences will appear.

As you read these vignettes, you may find they offer insights into your day-to-day experiences. While these stories might not capture your exact circumstance, you will most likely identify similar struggles and challenges. You can use these to validate that you are not alone in what you are experiencing, as well as creating your own recipe for what works best for you.

This is also a workbook. This book is highly practical with many points of reflection. It will be useful to come armed with a central place to record your reflections as you work through each chapter — either a pen and notebook, or have your computer handy.

At the end of each chapter, there are 'putting it into practice' reflection questions to help you adapt the content to your own unique situation. The 'getting the help you need' section is also full of handy points for reflection and learning.

You may want to pause and think through your own situation using the questions provided before moving on to the next chapter. You could even use these exercises as guidance to work through with your various practitioners.

Most of all, however you use this book, I want you to feel seen and understood at a time that can feel isolating and lonely. I want you to feel supported and know you are not alone, that there is a (sometimes twisted) pathway towards improvement and a new normal. Lastly, I want you to feel hope that you can learn to embrace your current reality and eventually navigate it. While recovery might not be exactly how you imagined, it can become about embracing a new normal that works for you.

I am about to share my pathway through fatigue, including the current phase of (tentatively hopeful) recovery, discovering my new normal.

So, pour yourself your favourite drink and sit (or lie) back as you dive straight into the first chapter — a framework for recovery.

Sarah Vizer

Chapter 1
A Framework for Recovery

Sarah's decline into fatigue came at age 40 after an unbelievably stressful period of life. She was first diagnosed with anxiety and depression. This diagnosis soon switched to burnout from her corporate life, later transitioning to chronic fatigue syndrome.

It was two years into Sarah's journey with fatigue that she started to accept she couldn't return to life as she knew it. Working long days in the corporate world was no longer possible, she did not have the energy to engage with friends and family like she used to, and social occasions were becoming few and far between.

She needed to let go of this Sarah from the past. The new Sarah? At first, it was a life she did not want to accept. She was living with a debilitating condition that the medical profession couldn't tell her much about. Some days she could barely drag herself out of bed. She often felt isolated and alone.

After a period of grief, a new way of thinking started to arise. Sarah began focusing just one day ahead, finding moments of enjoyment in her days. She stopped expecting so much from herself and started celebrating even the smallest signs of improvement. Relationships gradually became easier and new people entered her life.

This became a freeing way of thinking and kick-started a new chapter in Sarah's marathon journey of improvement and recovery.

Yes, I am the Sarah from that story! Many of us can relate long-term fatigue back to a virus, but for me it seemingly resulted from a period of unrelenting stress and corporate burnout.

Since researching burnout extensively, it's now quite obvious that I showed all the tell-tale signs — the exhaustion, the feelings of cynicism, the negativity and the low self-esteem. It was not fun, but the literature pointed to the fact that I could be confident life would go on and burnout would eventually resolve.

And it did resolve…in all ways but one. My exhaustion had set in. The part of my burnout story that was harder to get my mind around was the debilitating fatigue that seemed to not just take over my body, but affect every part of my being…mind, body and spirit.

It sometimes happens this way. Fatigue can be triggered by a virus or other illness — either explained or unexplained. It can also seemingly come from a life event. In my case, it was a build-up of toxic stress that led to my burnout event. High levels of stress over a long period of time can trigger all types of chronic health issues, and I now know that chronic fatigue is one of them.

This exhaustion stuck around long after all the other burnout symptoms went away. My mind healed and I was ready to move onto the next chapter of life, but my body could no longer keep up with this raring ambition.

Little did I know that I was about to enter the longest marathon event of my life — my journey of improvement and what I've termed 'recovery' (also known as creating a new normal).

Marathon of improvement and recovery

At the intersection of your physical, emotional and medical realities is your recovery process — a marathon effort towards improvement and eventually your recovery, or at least what I refer to as your 'new normal'.

The words 'improvement', 'recovery' and 'new normal' are used frequently throughout this book. While there is likely no fixed way of defining these terms, the following will give you some guideposts[10] as to what they involve:

- **Improvement** is defined as a substantial reduction in baseline symptoms, along with partial restoration of everyday activities with or without pacing or medication.
- **Full recovery** is defined as not experiencing post-exertional malaise (PEM) for six months and being able to perform what used to be your normal levels of activity without pacing or medication.
- **New normal** is defined as reaching a point of improvement where — while you do not experience full recovery in the truest sense and you still live with symptoms of fatigue — you have transformed your outlook on life compared to how you lived before your condition. You are effectively embracing a new reality, adapting life around the limitations of your condition.

---

10 Definitions for improvement and full recovery are loosely based on those provided in various studies conducted with ME/CFS patients.

As you navigate your journey throughout this book, I'd urge you to keep in mind that improvement and new normal are usually long-term processes that require your patience and stamina.

They are also non-specific endpoints, the exact timeline of which is unknown. If you look at case studies from those who have gone before you, the timeline for people experiencing substantial improvement vastly varies in length. With all the new treatment options being discovered, there is hope these pathways will eventually be drastically reduced, but for now living with long-term fatigue conditions can range from months to years.

Aside from not knowing when you're going to see improvement, it can also be a twisted pathway, full of ups and downs.

We often think the road to recovery should be steady progress over time, something like this:

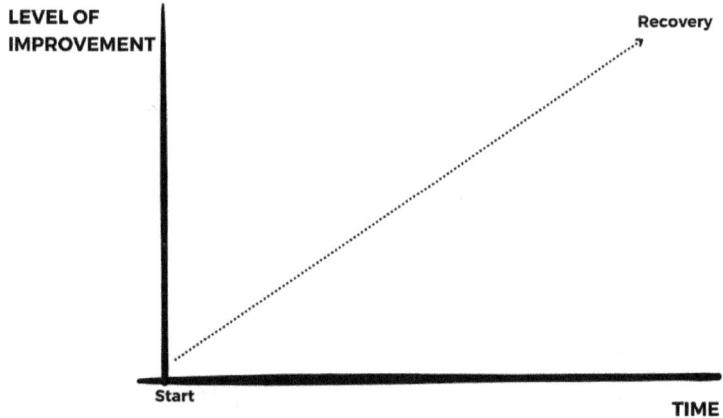

Figure 1 — Steady Progress to Recovery

Or it might be a long tail of symptoms, followed by a swift recovery period, such as this:

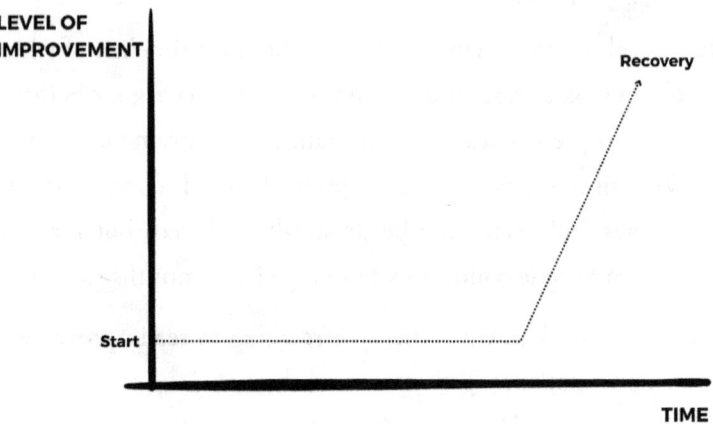

Figure 2 — Long Tail of Symptoms and Swift Recovery

For long-term fatigue, neither of these are accurate. Your marathon of improvement and recovery usually looks more like Figure 3 — a twisted pathway of peaks (improvements, celebration) and troughs (regression, disappointment).

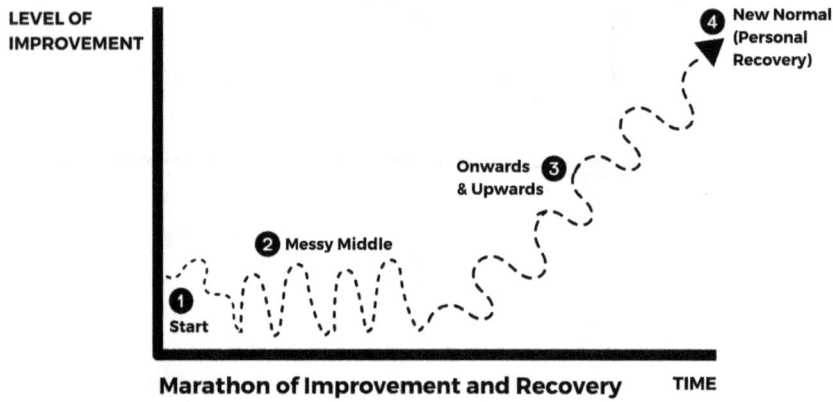

Figure 3 — Marathon of Improvement and Recovery

There are four stages we tend to navigate in the overall marathon:

1. Starting stage — something is wrong
2. Messy middle — peaks and troughs
3. Onwards and upwards — consistent improvement over time
4. New normal (personal recovery) — your new state of play

It is difficult to track every journey exactly and Figure 3 is only a rough estimation of how long-term fatigue can play out. Even if you can't relate to the whole journey, you will most likely relate to some of the stages.

Let's review these now so you can keep your current situation top of mind as you read through the rest of this book.

Stage 1 — Starting point...something is wrong

This is the start of your condition. In cases of post-viral fatigue, such as long-COVID, it's most likely easy enough to pinpoint when your symptoms first started. For ME/CFS and fibromyalgia, it might become more difficult to identify exactly when they began.

Often symptoms are vague, or they might worsen over time until you get to a point of being able to quantify that you do indeed have a fatigue condition. There is always the chance of misdiagnosis happening in between if your symptoms are attributed to a different condition.

At some point, you'll conclude that you have a condition resulting in fatigue and this brings with it a whole raft of rule and lifestyle changes.

The reality is the effects of fatigue are often invisible to other people. At my starting point, I didn't look unwell. My eyes were bright, my skin clear. I looked the picture of good health from all the different supplements my doctor had me taking. However, I was terribly affected. I just didn't have words for the gut-wrenching exhaustion I felt all the time. I was indeed too tired to think!

A previously conscientious and ambitious type of person, I was increasingly unable to cope with everyday demands. Out of necessity, I stripped away at life, cutting back, trying to make it more manageable. In the beginning, all I did was cut out the things that gave me pleasure. This left only work, a miserable place to be.

Eventually, I was forced to stop working altogether. I wasn't sleeping well and never felt refreshed, even though I slept all day. The things I used to get pleasure from became too hard. The people around me tried to understand, but how could they really? Their responses ranged from concern, to trying to motivate me, to leaving me alone as they didn't know what to do and I felt powerless to explain.

It took me a long time to answer the question: what is wrong with me? My starting point came six months after my fatigue condition first began when I finally heard the term 'chronic fatigue syndrome' from a health professional. This unlocked a pathway to understanding what I was dealing with, but there was limited information around what was going to heal me.

From this starting point comes your journey of peaks and troughs — what I like to call the messy middle.

Stage 2 — Messy middle…peaks and troughs

The messy middle is the perfect term for it as it is messy indeed. If you look at the pattern of our messy middle, the improvement pattern is not linear. It is a twisted path full of peaks (improvements, celebration), but also troughs (regression, disappointment).

In this stage, you are trying to pinpoint exactly what is occurring, looking for an accurate diagnosis. You are most likely seeking solid medical assistance, being tested to make sure your fatigue is not a sign of something more serious underneath.

With your diagnosis confirmed, you are then seeking the best forms of treatment. You might look for information from your medical team, books, support groups — anyone who can help you make sense of what is going on.

The time period for the messy middle is variable — it can last months or even years, challenging even the most resilient of us. It can feel like a never-ending endurance test. A marathon you undertake while feeling exhausted.

My messy middle was a four-year long struggle. I was seeing as many medical practitioners as I could manage on my limited energy. I focused on my health and worked as hard as my body allowed, but the fatigue was inside me, affecting every moment of life — waking and asleep. I felt like my body let me down time and time again as I tried to get back on track to the person I once was. Daily, my mind's ambition far outstripped my body's limited capability.

These were often lonely years as my friends and family struggled to understand my situation. When I gave my all, it only looked like 10% effort to those around me compared to my previous form. Some judged this harshly, I felt, even though this was actually my 100% effort. At times, it cost me a lot to even do this much. No matter how hard I tried to explain it to them, I frequently felt misunderstood. When you tell one person, and they react badly, you become reticent to tell the next. It's just easier to keep it all hidden.

There was a mix of good and bad over this time. The best thing throughout the messy middle was finding my pup Oliver. He was always at my side, motivating me to get out of bed and take him for walks, no matter what. His attitude was pure joy and he loved me to the exclusion of all else. Sometimes

I wonder if I'd even be here at all if it wasn't for Oliver; it always seemed like he understood, even when no one else could.

Another highlight of this time was meeting my partner Demian. Let this be a lesson that love can spring from the craziest of circumstances. Even when I was at my most fatigued, Demian could still see the burning energy inside me. To him, I was the most energetic person in the room. This felt like a gift of what I wanted most — to be seen and understood.

Over time, I started experiencing small signs of improvement that gradually became more regular. I could better hold a conversation as I had less brain fog. I started committing to events and could even make a few! I rejoiced after waking up feeling refreshed for the first time. My improvement trajectory was starting to trend upwards.

In your messy middle, you're most likely trying different things, with varying levels of success. At some point, you'll start to see signs of consistent improvement. What a relief! This is the beginning of the next stage of your journey.

Stage 3 — Onwards and upwards... consistent improvement over time

It can take time to notice your path is trending onwards and upwards. Gradually, your messy middle gives way to progress, and improvement in your symptoms feels consistent. Sometimes it's something you've done, or it could be that this improvement just happens with time.

It may be a result of medication or some other medical intervention. It may be better pacing yourself and diligently implementing lifestyle changes. You likely have a greater awareness of your limits and have adjusted your work and lifestyle accordingly. Sometimes you can't find a reason and don't know what to attribute it to other than time.

Whatever the reason, you are experiencing small, steady steps in improvement — you are on your way!

Four years into fatigue, my life started to show gradual consistent improvements. Slowly, I built on this until I reached a consistency in my energy levels that allowed me to trust in them again. Hallelujah, most days I was no longer too tired to think!

With more consistent energy, I learnt the art of chipping away at big projects. From small amounts of daily effort, big things can arise and my burnout program was born. I've also become a successful coach and consultant, gaining meaning from working with like-minded clients.

While I'm still affected by fatigue, I'm at a stage of recovery that I now accept as my new reality. At some point, you will also learn to accept life as it is, signalling the next stage and your new state of normality.

Stage 4 — New normal (personal recovery)... your new state of play

This last leg of the marathon is having a sense of your personal recovery, or what has become your new normal.

Full recovery implies you have fully healed from your long-term condition, no longer feeling any symptoms. For some, this means life returns to roughly how it was before you first had the experience of long-term fatigue. For many others, the length of time taken navigating this condition and the changes required in lifestyle and mindset result in some fundamental shifts. These might even be changes that you can look back on and feel have benefited you in some way.

I've heard many inspirational recovery stories over the years and feel great joy that this is indeed possible. I've also observed that a state of *absolute / I'm no longer affected / hallelujah I'm fully healed* recovery can be a difficult target to reach. To say you have absolutely no residual fatigue symptoms often only occurs after many, many years.

To this end, I've gradually subscribed to a different recovery reality, a bridging reality, which I call your 'new normal'.

New normal is a state of personal recovery where you may still live with fatigue symptoms and need to pace yourself. The difference is you have transformed your outlook on what life can be compared to before your condition, finding a level of peace and acceptance.

At my new normal, fatigue is still very much part of my reality. I feel the effects every day and need to pace myself. I'll occasionally cross the imaginary line where I do too much, only to face the exhausted blowback. I'm also highly aware of my limits and mostly find ways to stick to them. I'm once again working, albeit still on a part-time basis. I can regularly attend social events, plan travel adventures and make my difference in the world. The biggest change has been the ability to plan my day and know that I will stick to that plan. This is a sign of improvement that changed everything – what a gift it has been!

While it's the physical improvements that have allowed these changes, embracing your new normal is as much a mindset change as anything else. Your new normal might mean you've needed to change your lifestyle quite drastically, and this might not feel like recovery at all. I still feel frustrated, angry, even sad at times. However, I observe a growing sense of peace with this new reality; knowing that while my lifestyle has fundamentally changed and I can no longer live exactly how I used to, I can still enjoy a full, happy and productive life.

Once, I heard the line, '*Objects in the rear-view mirror will always appear better or worse than they actually were.*' When I look back at the process of accepting my new normal, chronic fatigue syndrome is both: it appears better as I'm a natural optimist who tends to gloss over the bad and focus on the good in life; it also appears worse as the level of pain, loneliness, isolation and sheer frustration of this time feels imprinted on my soul.

What will your new normal bring for you? Life in your new normal will be very much up to you. It will likely come with many lessons learnt, along with an altered way of viewing your world. A good question to ask yourself might be: '*What do I need in order to find peace and acceptance within my new reality?*'

Navigating your marathon journey

You will find the marathon model and four stages referred to at various points throughout the book. Knowing there are ups and downs, peaks and troughs, happiness and despair is an underlying assumption you can hold onto as you read through each chapter. This model aims to inspire flexibility in your mindset, knowing you are driving to a potential new normal outcome.

The last chapter also explores how best to manage your marathon journey and maintain perspective — a valuable skill for any challenging event in your life.

As you progress through the book, it's helpful to recognise that management of long-term fatigue is a complex process. The structure of distinct sections (physical, emotional, medical) has simplified what is in fact a much more intricate interplay.

Keep in mind they do not operate in a vacuum:

1. Being aware of what's going on in your own body helps you find the right medical care.

2. Your emotional experience overlays every aspect of your marathon journey.
3. Getting the right medical care helps you better understand and manage the physical effects.

I'd urge you to consider this as you read through each section, recognising how strongly the physical is tied to the emotional, which in turn influences your medical experience.

We start this journey with an exploration of the physical side to navigating long-term fatigue.

Physical Reality... Nurturing a Tired Body

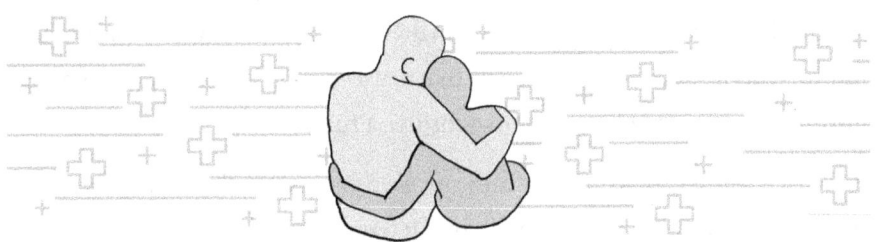

Scared and alone, people couldn't see what was going on inside me. To look at me, you wouldn't know anything had changed and I kept up a pretty good front. But my energy was almost non-existent, and I had a range of other symptoms that were difficult to explain. They didn't understand the loneliness, the pain, the self-doubt that resulted. How could they? What I was going through was mainly hidden and therefore difficult to recognise.

What is your physical reality? A typical day can be a challenge from the moment you wake up. People congratulate us when we do the big things in life, but some days even getting out of bed and having a shower *are* the achievement when you're dealing with long-term fatigue. Simple tasks like walking to the bathroom, removing your clothes, standing in the shower all require significant energy, leaving you feeling drained. It's rinse and repeat with all the other tasks that make up your days.

Understanding my physical reality took a long time to process — years even. It was a marathon event indeed! I was thrown by the lack of consensus within the medical community. I despaired that I would ever see substantial improvement, and no one flagged that I was potentially heading to a new normal rather than what I would consider a full recovery.

Eventually, I took matters into my own hands, my breakthrough coming when I stumbled across a book by Dr Sarah Myhill with the subtitle, '… it's mitochondria, not hypochondria'[11]. Catchy hey! Dr Myhill's work was considered 'fringe' at the time by many in the medical community, but it provided explanations as to what was going on with my body, including the 'holes in my energy bucket'. This book arrived at a time when I was finding any explanations of what was going on for me otherwise difficult to come by. Even today, many of us still struggle with the lack of consensus among the doctors who are meant to be helping us.

Understanding my physical reality was one thing; acceptance another. My tired body didn't fit who I knew myself to be, and I desperately tried any and all treatments that offered hope of redemption.

---

11   Dr Myhill's book is titled *Diagnosis and treatment of Chronic Fatigue Syndrome and Myalgic Encephalitis*. An interesting fact to note is Dr Myhill's choice to name the condition myalgic encephalitis not myalgic encephalomyelitis as it's more commonly referred to. The choice of terminology can vary, but some will argue that encephalomyelitis is more accurate as it reflects the involvement of both the brain (encephalo-) and spinal cord (myelo-). Reference: Myhill, Dr. Sarah (2017), *Diagnosis and treatment of Chronic Fatigue Syndrome and Myalgic Encephalitis*, Hammersmith Health Books.

I came to accept there was no short-cutting the process. Your tired body will heal in its own time. We can try all the things, but will eventually fall back on the tried-and-true methods of making our days as productive as possible while also getting the rest and recharge we so sorely need.

Buckle up because this section will consider the physical aspects of dealing with fatigue.

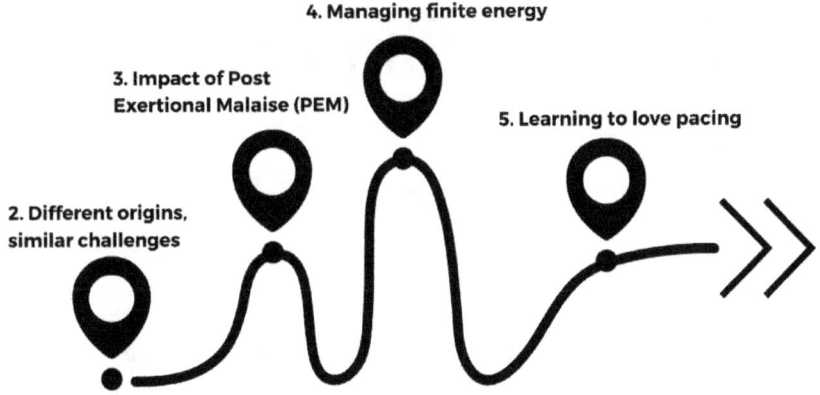

Figure 4 — Physical Reality Chapter Roadmap

- Symptoms of your fatigue condition, which we'll look at in Chapter 2.
- Energy challenges and methods of managing your finite energy in Chapters 3 and 4.
- Making the most of your days by implementing what is arguably *the* best treatment protocol in Chapter 5.

This is your physical reality: using the concept of energy over time management, pacing over your normal daily routine, and eventually acknowledging that a new normal has become your reality — at least for now.

Let's get started!

Chapter 2
Different Origins, Similar Challenges

Liam, a 46-year-old ex-police officer from just outside Winnipeg in Canada, has been diagnosed with ME/CFS. Liam needs to take it slow in the morning and on his worst days uses a wheelchair to get around his house. After a shower, he needs to rest again before breakfast and often feels light-headed. After breakfast, he has a short window of time to complete some light administration, walk slowly around the block or do some reading. Following this, he needs a significant rest period as his fatigue hits hard.

Liam will emerge again in the afternoon and often finds his mind quite foggy. After a career in the police force for 15 years, he finds the fogginess particularly difficult to accept as it's such a deviation from his normal persona. Lately, he's become shy around other people as he often forgets words or trails off mid-sentence. This is embarrassing to say the least and has been a catalyst for Liam to isolate himself from his friends and former colleagues.

During the afternoon, Liam will try to do some household chores, but finds even simple tasks — such as preparing a meal or doing laundry — can be tiring. Evenings are difficult, but he pushes himself to spend quality time with his family. He goes to bed around 8pm and often sleeps quite fitfully until he rises to start again the next day.

It's taken Liam a long time to understand what is happening to his body and accept his current schedule of activities. The isolation is wearing, and he still wishes he could maintain more sharpness of thinking and the stamina to do more around the house. Despite this, he has accepted this is his current reality for the time being.

What is meant by long-term fatigue? I've already hinted that fatigue is more than the day-to-day tiredness that everyone experiences. Tiredness after exertion, even exhaustion, is normal and not to be feared.

On the other hand, long-term fatigue is a debilitating condition and a misleading term compared to the severity of what people are experiencing. I often describe it as more like being hit by a truck! Others liken it to being on your feet all day, talking and burning brain power nonstop, then coming home and flopping on the couch. You're so exhausted you can't physically move, even to get yourself a glass of water, your whole body aching in tiredness. Imagine feeling this way *all the time* and you start to get the idea as to what fatigue feels like when it's long-term and critical.

Fatigue is considered long-term when it persists for an extended period, typically longer than six months. While the overarching symptom is extreme tiredness or exhaustion, rarely would this be the only symptom that you experience. It is usually accompanied by a wide array of other symptoms[12], some of which can even be diagnosed as conditions themselves.

---

12 ME/CFS and fibromyalgia are usually accompanied by a range of symptoms; we look at the most common ones experienced. However, long-COVID is another level! At last count, the World Health Organisation has identified over 200 symptoms that may accompany long-COVID.

What is common is this pervasive exhaustion that is not relieved by rest or sleep. When you are experiencing long-term fatigue, you feel this exhaustion daily, inevitably leading to difficulty performing everyday activities. You can see from Liam's example in the snapshot above that it can affect even the simplest of tasks, such as cooking, taking a shower or having a simple conversation. Fatigue can range in severity from affecting a few hours of the day to requiring complete bed rest most of the time.

Overview of fatigue conditions

Long-term fatigue arises from complex conditions, resulting in difficulties with explanations and diagnosis. As a result, they are often widely misunderstood — by the person experiencing the condition, their friends, family, work and (really worryingly) the medical community.

This book has been specifically written for you if you are dealing with long-term fatigue within three conditions.

1. **Myalgic encephalomyelitis/chronic fatigue syndrome** (otherwise known as ME/CFS) is characterised by severe, persistent fatigue, with symptoms that worsen with physical and mental activity, and don't fully improve with rest[13].
   ME/CFS is a complex medical condition that is still poorly understood. There is no specific test for this condition and a diagnosis is usually made by considering a combination of symptoms and ruling out other medical conditions.

2. **Fibromyalgia** is a disorder of the central nervous system characterised by chronic widespread musculoskeletal pain and joint swelling. It is commonly accompanied by fatigue and can also coexist with a range of

---

13 Based on the Mayo Clinic definition of ME/CFS at www.mayoclinic.org

other issues, including non-refreshing sleep, generalised stiffness, headaches, irritable bowel syndrome and irritable bladder, cold sensitivity, restless legs, exercise intolerance, and memory and mood issues[14].

It can coexist with ME/CFS. In fact, one of the major issues people face with this condition is long-term fatigue, often thought to arise from the energy expenditure in the management of pain and insufficient sleep[15].

3. **Long-COVID** stems from SARS-CoV-2 (COVID-19) infections. It is defined as a continuation or development of new symptoms three months after the initial COVID-19 infection, with these symptoms lasting for at least two months with no other explanation[16].

Long-COVID sufferers, also called long-haulers, are often diagnosed with ME/CFS as part of their condition. The long-COVID community has frequently turned to the ME/CFS community for advice in managing this condition.

The commonalities within these three conditions are they all have the potential to result in ME/CFS type symptoms. They are frequently also accompanied by mood issues such as depression and anxiety, often in response to management of these long-term chronic conditions.

Despite these commonalities, the symptoms experienced within these conditions themselves can be vastly different. For example, two people with long-COVID can experience different sets of symptoms, different recovery

---

14 List compiled based on the work by Dr David Brady, an expert in fibromyalgia. His work encompasses 'The Fibro Fix', a book dedicated to addressing the treatment of fibromyalgia. You can find out more from his website: drdavidbrady.com
15 Healthline article dated 7 January 2022 outlines the relationship between fibromyalgia and fatigue. According to the National Fibromyalgia Association, around 76% of fibromyalgia sufferers experience fatigue that does not go away even after sleep or rest. Article link — www.healthline.com/health/fibromyalgia/fibromyalgia-fatigue#seeking-help
16 This long-COVID definition has been taken from the World Health Organization site, where studies indicate 10 to 20% of people infected with COVID-19 may go on to develop long-COVID. Please note that what we know about long-COVID continues to evolve. Other sources suggest that long-COVID can be present after as little as four to six weeks of symptoms.

rates and different treatment effectiveness. It's counterintuitive in so many ways!

When accounting for these differences in how fatigue presents itself, I've kept the content of this book as general as possible. You will not find a laundry list of symptoms or treatment options as this would be an ever-changing landscape. Instead, the focus is on broad concepts that invite you to rise above the detail when reading. You can think about the management of your condition holistically, along with where to get help with your own more specific treatment options.

I've written this book so that even if you don't fit neatly in one of the above categories or conditions, or you don't yet have a diagnosis, but fatigue is an issue, you will still benefit from the many tools in this book.

Understanding fatigue and managing life, emotions and energy levels is highly valuable for **those with other long-term chronic conditions** as well. If you are someone who can't operate at 100% all day every day, you may face similar challenges to those described and find many points here that resonate.

In addition, there are numerous other causes of long-term fatigue that have not been specifically considered when writing this book, where people may also face similar challenges[17].

These include:

- **Chronic medical conditions** such as autoimmune diseases, diabetes, thyroid conditions, multiple sclerosis, lupus, cancer.

---

17 The Mayo Clinic offers a comprehensive list of conditions that feature 'exhaustion that doesn't let up' as a symptom. Site link — www.mayoclinic.org/symptoms/fatigue/basics/causes/sym-20050894

- **Functional disorders** such as anaemia, gastrointestinal imbalance of the gut microbiome and toxicity, other infections such as Lyme disease, Ross River fever, EpsteinBarr virus, or dysglycemia (insulin resistance present without a diabetes diagnosis).
- **Mental health conditions** such as depression (major depressive disorder or clinical depression), grief, anxiety disorders, stress or physical or emotional abuse.
- **Sleep disorders** such as sleep apnoea and insomnia.
- **Lifestyle factors** such as poor diet, obesity, alcohol or drug use, lack of or too much exercise, or exposure to environmental toxins.

What is apparent is that regardless of the origin of long-term fatigue, individuals often face similar challenges.

Even if you haven't been diagnosed formally, you still might find much of the commentary resonates. I'm excited by the wider benefit this book can provide, including strategies that will help improve the situation of anyone struggling with long-term fatigue. No matter how this relates to you, you're very welcome here too.

Symptoms to expect

Liam's example in the opening snapshot demonstrates a common issue — fatigue symptoms can be frustratingly vague. Foggy thinking, forgetting words, tired after engaging in easy chores, feeling light-headed from a shower — what a weird set of symptoms!

Anyone living with long-term fatigue will most likely experience a wide array of these symptoms, significantly impacting their quality of life. Sometimes these are a sign of a more serious underlying medical condition, and your medical team should rule this out as a first response. Other times there is seemingly no logical reason for what you are experiencing.

If fatigue does not arise from an underlying condition, it can be identified as either the main symptom you are experiencing or classified as the condition in itself. This is where the fun starts! Deciphering these symptoms can be a nightmare effort and anyone who has had fatigue long enough will tell you it can be notoriously difficult to diagnose and manage.

It can be hit or miss as to whether your medical team can help you make sense of the symptoms you are experiencing. With viral conditions like long-COVID, it can usually be traced back to the original infection. With conditions like ME/CFS and fibromyalgia, the origin of fatigue can be less understood. Complications arise when you don't first relate the symptoms you are experiencing to your long-term fatigue condition.

Let's start here — gaining a better understanding of the symptoms you are experiencing. The following checklist is not exhaustive, but rather lists the more commonly experienced symptoms that most often accompany long-term fatigue.

Note: *There is a wide array of symptoms reported with viral conditions like long-COVID, up to 200 at last count*[18].

---

18 The World Health Organization references reports of over 200 different long-COVID symptoms that impact everyday functioning. If unsure about the symptoms you're experiencing as part of long-COVID, seeking expert advice from your doctor or a specialised long-COVID clinic may help you understand the full extent of your particular set of symptoms.

Tick all the symptoms you are currently experiencing or have previously experienced in the checklist below.

- [x] **Fatigue** – Feelings of persistent and overwhelming lack of energy and exhaustion that is not alleviated by rest or sleep. It is often accompanied by physical and mental weariness and interferes with daily functioning and activities.

- [ ] **Post Exertional Malaise (PEM)** – After-effects of physical, mental, or emotional exertion. These effects can last for hours, even days and often leads to prolonged exhaustion, brain fog, and other debilitating symptoms.

- [ ] **Brain fog** - Cognitive difficulties that can feel like a layer of fogginess overlaying your thinking. This leads to issues with memory, your ability to concentrate, and decision-making capability.

- [ ] **Body aches** - Various types of body pain, including joint pain, muscle pain, headaches, and migraines.

- [ ] **Gastrointestinal problems** – Issues such as nausea, bloating, constipation, and diarrhoea.

- [ ] **Dizziness / vertigo** – Light-headedness, feeling like you might faint, feeling off balance, and sensations of spinning or moving.

- [ ] **Sleep issues** – Varied issues such as not getting good sleep and carrying a sleep debt throughout the day, waking up feeling unrefreshed or sleeping at odd times during the day and not being able to sleep well at night.

- [ ] **Mood Impacts** – Feeling negative emotions such as irritability, frustration, sadness, loneliness, depression, and anxiety.

- [ ] **Postural Orthostatic Tachycardia Syndrome (POTS)** – A medical condition characterised by abnormal increases in heart rate when in an upright position. Often results in symptoms such as light-headedness, fainting, and feelings of weakness.

Table 1 — Fatigue Symptom Checker

The symptom checker provides you with a big-picture view of the symptoms you are experiencing. Some of these symptoms are self-explanatory; others warrant a deeper look and more explanation. Let's look more closely at the characteristics and examples of the lesser understood symptoms, some of which may even be classified as conditions in themselves.

Post-exertional malaise (PEM)

This is the after-effects of physical, mental or emotional exertion. PEM can be triggered by even minor exertion. PEM effects will arise based on varied timelines, ranging from hours or even several days after exertion, and can last for hours, days or even weeks at a time.

Physical effects of PEM include:
- Fatigue
- Muscle weakness
- Joint pain
- Headaches
- Dizziness or light-headedness
- Flu-like symptoms, such as fever, chills and sore throat
- Increased heart rate or heart palpitations
- Nausea or gastrointestinal symptoms
- Sensitivity to light and sound

Mental effects of PEM include:
- Cognitive dysfunction, also known as 'brain fog'
- Difficulty concentrating or remembering things
- Slower information processing
- Reduced attention span
- Poor decision-making and problem-solving abilities
- Mental exhaustion

Emotional effects of PEM include:
- Anxiety or nervousness
- Depression or low mood
- Irritability or mood swings
- Emotional exhaustion or burnout
- Reduced motivation or interest in activities
- Social isolation or withdrawal

PEM is so prevalent and such an important part of managing long-term fatigue that Chapter 3 is dedicated entirely to this topic!

PEM in action:

> *"Last week, I met up with my brother and we did a 3km walk. I've had long-COVID for six months now and this walk was mostly flat and one that we did regularly with ease before I had COVID-19. I wasn't thinking too hard and just enjoying his company, but I guess I pushed past the amount of activity that had become my norm. Two hours later the effects of this one walk had me feeling weak, nauseated and with severe brain fog. I was exhausted the next day and developed a headache. These effects lasted for the next three days, during which I was basically laid up in bed or on the couch for the whole time."*

In another case:

> *"I went out with some close family members and had an amazing three-hour lunch. I really needed it as it had been so long since I'd had any social interaction. My ME/CFS symptoms had been a lot milder lately, so I thought it would be okay. But later that night, I felt like I'd been hit by a semi-trailer! My body ached all over and I knew that I had overdone it. It scared me a bit, but looking back overall it was worth the*

bonding time. Next time I might limit my social time to an hour and a half maximum."

Brain fog

Brain fog is the user-friendly way of saying you are having difficulty thinking. Often called cognitive disfunction, it is quite an apt description as it feels like a layer of fogginess that settles over your thinking. You might feel disconnected, like there is a pane of glass between you and the world. I've even heard it being described as 'like being hungover, minus the fun!'

This fogginess results in a range of effects including difficulty concentrating, poor memory, trouble finding words and forming sentences, immediately forgetting new information, feeling confused, feeling spaced out and detached, forgetting how to do simple things and difficulty making decisions. Some of the symptoms might even be similar to conditions such as dementia, memory loss or ADHD.

At its worst, you may struggle with even the simplest of tasks that require focus or retention of information. Brain fog is where the name of this book comes from — *Too Tired to Think*. I experience this feeling daily throughout the afternoon and into the evening. It's the days you wake up with clarity of thought, where the fog seems to lift for a while, that reveal just how much the fog impacts your ability to think!

Brain fog in action:

> *"It was evening and we needed cat food, so I went out to the nearest place that was open and ended up bringing back a bag of cat litter! Not to be beaten, the next day I was determined to get the cat food and asked a friend for a lift to the store. When we got home, I realised I'd forgotten…you guessed it, the cat food! I did get some nice cheese though."*

In another case:

> "My sister is getting married in Queensland, Australia. I live around 500km away and am desperate to attend. She's been so accommodating and offering some great suggestions on how to make the trip easier on me, but my brain fog is making it so difficult to make decisions. She's giving me lots of choices to make; honestly, all I want is for someone else to make the decisions and do the planning on my behalf!"

Sleep issues

Sleep issues can be many and varied with long-term fatigue. Your sleep patterns might be all over the place — sleeping during the day and then up all night. It can be you have difficulty falling asleep in the first place or have trouble staying asleep at night even when you are extremely tired.

Then there is the torturous practice of sleeping through the night but waking up feeling unrefreshed. You might then feel exhausted and sleep at odd hours during the day, doomed to fall back into the pattern of not being able to sleep at night. I often need to sleep during the day, but find myself so tired that even lying down to sleep brings no relief; rather it feels difficult and exhausting.

Some people also report night terrors, a sleep disorder with sudden episodes of intense fear, terror or dread during sleep.

All these patterns have been reported by others with long-term fatigue. Not getting enough good quality sleep serves to add exponentially to the tiredness and brain fog you feel during the day.

Sleep issues in action:

> *"Getting restful sleep is a nightmare for me (pun intended!). I go to bed early and sleep well into the next morning. I wake feeling unrefreshed. Sometimes it feels like I'm just as tired as when I first went to bed despite being in bed for a good 12 hours."*

Postural orthostatic tachycardia syndrome (POTS)

POTS is a form of dysautonomia affecting the autonomic nervous system, which regulates involuntary bodily functions such as heart rate, blood pressure and digestion[19]. POTS involves a significant increase in heart rate when standing up (tachycardia) and other symptoms such as:

- Dizziness or light-headedness
- Shaking and sweating
- Weakness and fatigue
- Shortness of breath
- Chest pain
- Fainting
- Heart palpitations
- Headaches
- Poor sleep

It can be triggered by as little as walking up a set of stairs and other factors such as dehydration, prolonged bed rest and certain medications.

POTS can be serious, and it is important to seek medical assistance for an accurate diagnosis and appropriate treatment plan. Wearable technology such as a smart watch or Fitbit can be helpful for gathering data to help di-

---

[19] POTS UK is a great site for visually understanding more about POTS, the symptoms and how to manage the condition. Find this at www.potsuk.org

agnose this condition, such as resting heart rate and heart rate changes when standing and moving.

POTS in action:

> *"I was experiencing random bouts of a racing pulse and heart rate spikes during the day, even when I was just sitting on the sofa. It felt like adrenaline rushes and then came the tiredness. I measured it all on my smart watch and tried to find out what was going on. The first doctor I saw dismissed it as an anxiety diagnosis. The second doctor was better — actually running some tests and helping me understand that what I was experiencing was POTS."*

In another case:

> *"I found I was really affected by POTS when I had to stand still for any length of time. Standing in queues, even trying to visit the shops would result in getting out of breath, pulse racing, dizzy spells and shaking muscles. It got to the point where I could no longer stand. There was one time when I could barely make it back to my car and I had to lie down in the back until I could drive myself home."*

What symptoms have you experienced?

Fatigue is the common denominator, but you're most likely now realising how often it is accompanied by a range of other symptoms that impact your day-to-day and lead to that tired body of yours.

One of the frustrating aspects of long-term fatigue is there is no one set of symptoms that you can treat. The type and severity of symptoms you experience will be individual to your situation. There may even have been symptoms on that list that you had not even recognised as being part of your condition!

One symptom that is critically important in the diagnosis and treatment of fatigue is PEM. Next is a deep dive into understanding the triggers of PEM and the impact of boom-and-bust cycles that you may be experiencing.

Putting it into practice

This is where you can really start to understand your fatigue symptoms and even use the symptom checker as a tool to take to your next medical appointment.

First you will need somewhere to write — a new document, a clean sheet of paper, a book or a journal.

Refer back to the checklist on page 37 for all the fatigue symptoms you have ticked and write down more detail. If you can remember, record the frequency of symptoms, when they occur, how long they've been occurring for, what triggers each symptom and anything else that feels relevant. Include any other symptoms not mentioned in the checklist that you can also relate to your condition.

Chapter 3
The Impact of Post-Exertional Malaise

Priya is a 29-year-old stockbroker living in New York. In mid 2022 she contracted what seemed like a mild case of COVID-19 but found her energy levels crashed after her initial recovery. She could hardly function from day to day.

Priya had been in intense training for the November 2022 New York Marathon. After a two-week break, she started to feel okay again and resumed work and training. After a week back at it, she found herself crashing again with intense fatigue, muscle and joint pain and a splitting headache. She gave herself a few more days to recover.

This cycle of crashing and recovery continued, with the time between crashes becoming shorter each time. Priya continued trying to train in her recovery times until she felt so unwell that she had to make the decision to pull out of the marathon altogether. Being such a strong and motivated person, making this decision hurt more than the actual illness!

> *During this time, her doctor ran a whole gamut of tests, and her bloodwork came back within normal ranges. Eventually she was diagnosed with long-COVID, including severe PEM. She was advised to stop her training altogether. This was a shocking and debilitating time for Priya, and she remains unsure as to when she will be able to resume her normal level of activity.*

PEM is such a significant but misunderstood symptom that I feel it warrants its own chapter. It is usually central to the diagnosis for any long-term fatigue condition.

In simple terms, PEM is the after-effects of physical or mental exertion. It occurs when your energy envelope — or the amount of energy you have available each day — is exceeded. Go too hard one day and you experience consequences that can last for hours, days or even weeks. These after-effects also vary when they occur, often delayed by several hours or even days. After-effects can be triggered by a lot of activity, or even simple tasks like having a shower or reading.

PEM feels like a crash, a relapse or a collapse. With this crash comes the resurgence of the other symptoms of fatigue — the body pain, weakness, muscle pain, headaches, nausea, cognitive difficulties, brain fog and an overwhelming exhaustion that rest will just not fix.

Literature from those who don't understand PEM describe it in terms such as 'general malaise'. This is such a polite term and can come across as being quite condescending, even victim-blaming. The actual effect is more like going ten rounds with a heavyweight boxer! PEM is your big, flashing warning sign, saying you've done too much.

Despite how obvious it can be that you've overdone it, PEM can still be so difficult to manage. Like Priya, our stockbroker from New York in the opening snapshot, so many of us with long-term fatigue are affected by

PEM. Priya developed a cycle of train hard, crash, rest and recover, train hard, crash again, take even more time to rest and recover. This became a perpetual cycle until she was forced to quit her training altogether — an emotionally devastating decision to have to make, I'm sure.

What Priya is demonstrating is a common experience, often referred to as boom-and-bust cycles.

Boom-and-bust cycles

For so many people, we are habitually emptying our energy envelope, leading to a cycle of boom-and-bust. This refers to a pattern where we are expending large amounts of energy over a short period of time (boom), followed by necessary rest or inactivity to recover (bust).

This is relevant for everyone! It has become common to follow this cycle in life, no matter your fatigue levels. You might have a large project at work or an event such as a wedding to organise. You push yourself hard to complete all you need to do, working long hours, focusing on little else and expending significant amounts of our energy doing so. Once the project is complete, the wedding is done or the event is over, you can rest. This often involves crashing for several days or even weeks for an intense recovery period.

What's different when you are living with long-term fatigue is that it can be a **perpetual cycle of boom-and-bust** — constantly pushing yourself to get through the day and complete all the activity you need to do, exhausting your daily energy envelope, then crashing to recover from this level of activity. You can recover just enough, but never actually feel like you are fully restoring enough energy to stop the cycle.

Priya in the opening snapshot demonstrated a classic boom-and-bust cycle as she tried in vain to keep up with her training for the New York Marathon. Her cycle of crashing and recovery — with the time between crashes becoming shorter after each crash — is a common experience. The cycle itself can be utterly debilitating to say the least.

It's not always those with high activity levels who fall into the boom-and-bust pattern either. When you are living with long-term fatigue, the boom-and-bust cycle might come from minimal amounts of activity, but result in the same outcome nonetheless.

Some examples of the boom-and-bust cycle include:

- You're trying to balance work and life with long-term fatigue, resulting in you spending all your energy on work. You crash straight after work and also on weekends, having little left over for other aspects of life, such as maintaining social connections, regular exercise or cooking healthy meals. This becomes an unhealthy and lonely experience.
- You're competitive and motivated, regularly competing in events such as marathons or triathlons. Long-term fatigue can be difficult to accept, so you try to continue your training through the fatigue, resulting in intense crashes and rest periods. Bitter frustration always seems to follow.
- You're feeling inspired and motivated by a certain project (such as writing a book!) and you push yourself to complete the task, ignoring the fatigue warnings. The result is an intense crash to be endured until you have the energy to return to your project again, inspiration still going strong.

For me, as I was adjusting to life with chronic fatigue syndrome and my new normal, I was caught by this boom-and-bust cycle over and over again. I pushed the boundaries — trying to keep up work, go to my social engagements and attend all my medical appointments to find answers. Even activities like reading a book at home seemed to have after-effects. Any conversation where I felt emotional or watching sad or stressful movies triggered debilitating fatigue.

The hardest aspect of all was the invisible line that I was never quite sure when I might cross. This line seemed to move daily. The minute I crossed this line, accidently or knowingly, there was a price to be paid. Depending on how hard I'd gone, that price could result in being laid up for hours or even days. Sometimes I handled it. Other times it felt devastating.

This invisible line is shared by anyone who experiences PEM. It can be one of the most difficult and frustrating aspects of managing long-term fatigue. It can seem impossible to decipher a pattern within our varying energy ebbs and flows. The fact that PEM can also be delayed by days can make it tricky to estimate if and when it will arise from activities in your schedule.

You can experience PEM at any of the four stages of your marathon journey, but it is usually particularly pervasive as you navigate your messy middle and the onwards and upwards stages. You may even experience PEM as part of your new normal if you tend to overdo things from time to time.

I still experience PEM as part of my new normal as I haven't yet learnt the meaning of the word 'moderation'! This tendency has become a blessing and a curse, pushing me to achieve incredibly ambitious projects such as writing this book, but also causing distress when I inevitably overdo it and face the resulting exhaustion. It's an ongoing journey — one I hope to help you navigate more easily!

What triggers PEM?

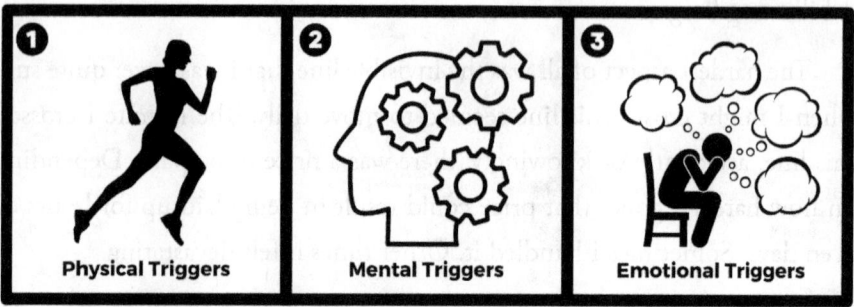

Figure 5 — Methods of Triggering PEM

PEM is all about overexertion — exhausting your energy envelope. When you think about this, what comes to mind? Most likely, you will identify physical triggers, such as physical activity or exercise. But it's not just the after-effects from movement that creates PEM and our boom-and-bust cycle. It's also from the mental or cognitive and emotional loads we shoulder as well.

What triggers PEM will differ from person to person. It can be anything that stresses or taxes your nervous system, subtle or extreme. These lists are not exhaustive, but the big-ticket triggers of PEM that have been reported include the following physical, mental and emotional triggers.

Tick all the triggers you are currently experiencing (or have previously experienced) in the following checklist.

PHYSICAL PEM TRIGGERS

- [ ] Physical exertion or exercise, such as walking, running, or lifting weights
- [ ] Overexertion during daily activities, such as household chores or work-related tasks
- [ ] Prolonged periods of standing or sitting in the same position
- [ ] Exposure to extreme temperatures, such as heat or cold
- [ ] Lack of sleep or poor sleep quality
- [ ] Travelling long distances or changing time zones
- [ ] Illness or infection, even if it's a mild one like a cold or flu
- [ ] Inflammation or pain in the body, such as from a flare-up of a chronic condition
- [ ] Allergies or sensitivities to food or environmental factors

MENTAL PEM TRIGGERS

- [ ] Concentrating for a period, such as reading, writing, driving, or watching children
- [ ] Mental problem-solving or decision-making
- [ ] Multi-tasking or frequently switching between tasks
- [ ] Sensory overload, such as being in a noisy or crowded location
- [ ] Overstimulation from electronic devices, such as computer screens or smartphones
- [ ] Exposure to bright lights or loud sounds
- [ ] Processing complex information or learning new things
- [ ] Social interactions or communication, such as speaking or listening intently.

EMOTIONAL PEM TRIGGERS

- [ ] Stress or anxiety, including worrying about future events or deadlines
- [ ] Intense emotions, such as anger, sadness, or excitement
- [ ] Social interactions, such as attending social events or interacting with others
- [ ] Sensitivity to emotional content in movies, books, or other media
- [ ] Overthinking or rumination, particularly about negative or distressing events
- [ ] Trauma or past experiences that may be triggered by current events or circumstances
- [ ] Lack of emotional support or feeling isolated

Table 2 — PEM Triggers Checklist

What triggers PEM for you?

As you can see, there are so many triggers to PEM that you may not have been aware of before. If you combine more than one of these triggers, such as being out at an event (which may already feel quite physical), and you also find yourself in a tense conversation, or feel it's too noisy and crowded, this only serves to intensify the triggers and after-effects.

Although you have these lists of triggers, it is also important to note that PEM can be present just from resting for those in the throes of long-term fatigue. It's a wily opponent indeed!

The challenge becomes understanding your own energy envelope — or your available energy —and the pattern of when PEM will occur. You can use the lists above to start looking for your own triggers.

- Is it physical and about the amount of activity you take on?
- Is it emotional or stressful situations?
- Do emotional or stressful movies or TV shows feel draining?
- Do you get decision fatigue being overloaded by the number of decisions you make daily?
- Are you trying to work or read for too long a period and need shorter sessions?
- Are you spiralling and your negative thoughts are becoming overwhelming?
- Could it be a lack of good quality sleep?

Maybe you're just in an intense period and you're going to experience PEM no matter what you do!

My earlier experiences with PEM still give me a horrified shiver when I think about them. Doing my weekly shopping online, a short walk with my pup, or even a quick 10-minute phone call could be enough to wipe me out for the rest of my day. Add in anything emotionally taxing to this mix and I was cactus for days[20]!

Medical appointments were particularly gruelling, as they required me to think and communicate clearly. They often also *really* wound me up, particularly when the practitioner was not 'chronic fatigue friendly', or had no idea about what I was going through. For these reasons, I tried to schedule only one appointment a week.

For those experiencing long-term fatigue, PEM is truly one of the hardest aspects to deal with — not just the physical aspects, but the emotional side as well.

One of the aims for managing long-term fatigue is to establish what consistent level of activity you can maintain over time, considering the physical, mental and emotional loads you carry.

This involves establishing a regular routine of activity — e.g. work, exercise, self-care, rest, social — that works to your energy levels and minimises PEM. For some, they find this is very low, and activity is very basic. For others, they can find a level of activity that works well with their lifestyle. The amount and type of activity you can sustain will change as you traverse your different marathon stages.

Over time, you may start to feel improvement and become able to add more activity into your day. I've slowly built up my tolerance to activity over the years. I still have instances where PEM catches me by surprise; however, these have become rare.

- I know my physical, mental and emotional triggers.

---

20 'Cactus for days' is Australian for I was basically really, really, really, really tired for the rest of the week! This is PEM at its finest.

- I've learnt how to realistically schedule my weeks, accounting for my current energy levels.
- I listen to my body and (most of the time!) only do the activities that I know I can do in that week.
- I've accepted this is a good life and appreciate my chances to rest and recharge!

Most of all, I've established a routine of activity that allows me to achieve within my new normal pace of life. The way to establish a routine of activity that works for your energy levels is called pacing, a hugely important concept in managing long-term fatigue.

Next, we examine the concept of finite energy, which will help you quantify just how much activity you can tolerate in your day. It's all about making choices that are in your own best interests — quantifying your fatigue and understanding more about your fluctuations in energy levels.

Putting it into practice

Take a moment to identify your experiences with PEM.

1. What does the boom-and-bust cycle look like for you?
2. Have you noticed an invisible line that leads to PEM when crossed?
3. What are your physical, mental and emotional triggers for PEM?
4. Can you see a pattern of events, activities or situations that lead to PEM being most likely to occur?

Chapter 4
Managing Finite Energy

Anna is a 30-year-old bakery assistant in Paris who has been living with ME/CFS for the past three years. Her typical day starts with waking up feeling exhausted, despite having slept for 10 hours. She gets ready slowly and makes her way to work.

Anna has negotiated a part-time arrangement at a local patisserie, but often finds it difficult to focus and must take frequent breaks throughout the day. The patisserie where she works has busy and quiet periods, so her employer allows rest and breaks during quieter times, which keeps the pace of working mostly manageable.

After work, Anna finds she has little energy left for socialising or leisure activities and usually spends her evenings resting at home with Bonbon, her Persian cat. On her days off, Anna has decided the best way to spend her energy is enjoying quality time with family and friends. While she finds this takes a lot out of her physically, she enjoys an emotional boost from her time with loved ones. She feels it's worth the trade-off of this heart boost versus the inevitable crash she feels afterwards.

Wouldn't we all love to have endless energy all the time? When we're young — a child or young adult — it may seem that we have infinite energy with no limitation or thought required.

I've always been a high-energy person, seemingly with energy to burn. I loved keeping busy and was always ready for the next thing to launch myself into, often with no thought to the consequences. Sometimes I was tired, but aware of this and able to recharge at night and on weekends. However, I had very little skill in the art of energy management.

One day when I hit my forties, I needed these energy management skills — almost overnight! I was working in a career I loved, but had found increasingly stressful over the years. It was this chronic, grinding stress that finally overtook my life, leaving me physically exhausted, mentally scattered and emotionally distraught.

I experienced deep tiredness everywhere in my body, not unlike wading through deep water and feeling the ocean current pulling you down. This was more than my normal tiredness; every cell in my body ached with an exhaustion I had never felt before. It was present no matter how much I tried to rest and recharge. I've mentioned previously that this book was almost called *Too Tired to Rest* — a good descriptor for this exhaustion.

Day by day, it worsened until it seemed like everything was draining me. Every interaction. Every responsibility I normally handled with ease. This became more than just about work/life balance. I was struggling to maintain any kind of social life. Even the basics, such as grocery shopping and keeping my house clean, became a struggle. I was ruminating at night and waking up feeling just as tired as when I first went to sleep. The book title came to life — I was literally too tired to think!

I tried to ignore it, holding onto my normal routine for far too long. The physical, mental and emotional effects snowballed until I could no longer hold down my job and was forced to take leave. What started as temporary leave turned into a permanent resignation. By then, I was irreversibly in a state of complete exhaustion and long-term fatigue had set in.

Only then, after it felt like I'd lost everything, was I diagnosed with chronic fatigue syndrome. It was from this state of exhaustion and a shock diagnosis that I took a crash course in energy management. Coming from the corporate world, I was used to being able to manage my time, but managing my energy was a completely foreign concept. I also didn't have the energy to invest in learning these vital skills. Not the ideal scenario!

My story is so often how it occurs. Just like Anna in the opening snapshot, so many of us in the prime of our life are suddenly very affected by post-viral fatigue or a fatigue that seemingly invades out of nowhere. Instantly, we must modify our whole life around its effects. This can be one of the most difficult elements of this condition — learning to manage our day with a new set of rules that govern our energy.

Energy management — your new set of rules into action

Energy management has become a helpful concept and life skill that has arisen from of my time with chronic fatigue syndrome. It's an incredibly important topic to get your head around and will provide benefit for everyone you share it with, not just those of us with long-term fatigue. You saw that I learnt this skill later in life and from a place of exhaustion that was not ideal. The more proactive you can be in managing your energy, the more sustainable life becomes.

Let's start by evaluating your current energy situation. Long-term fatigue covers a lot of ground with many different conditions that lead to it.

Your current energy situation will depend on the stage you are at with your condition.

- You might still be in the thick of it and very affected.
- You might find your energy is picking up, but you still need to be cautious about what you do in your day.
- You might be at the end of your journey and on a good path to recovery, or at least working within your new normal.

No matter what, you will most likely also experience regular fluctuations in your energy envelope, based on your symptom triggers and the amount of PEM you experience. These fluctuations can make it extremely difficult to estimate what your daily experience is going to be, varying from good energy one day and crashing the next.

Let's consider an easy method that I use to assess my own current energy envelope. It is basically assigning a number to your baseline level of energy for the day, out of a possible 10. Assessing energy levels is never an absolute value, so I call this my energy continuum to reflect the ever-changing nature of our energy profiles.

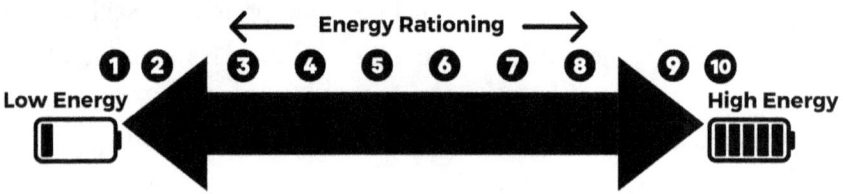

Figure 6 — Energy Continuum

Each day, you can assess your energy level on the continuum, assigning a number out of a possible 10. Once you have this, you can use the following points of reference to assess what that day holds.

Low energy (1 or 2 out of 10) — The amount of energy you have when your battery is low. You might be virtually bed-bound with small amounts of movement tolerated. Use of a wheelchair might be required. Simple activities such as getting up and showering require rest afterward.

Energy rationing (anywhere between 3 to 8 out of 10) — In between low and high energy, you have a certain amount of energy to use in the day. You might have less energy than is required to work full-time, but enough to do common household tasks, take short walks outside, etc. Completing activities often requires rest afterwards and too much exertion results in PEM.

High energy (9 or 10 out of 10) — The amount of energy you have when your battery is at full charge. 'Normal' activities are possible, such as work, social occasions and exercise and you do not get PEM after completing these activities.

Where are you right now on your energy continuum?

The continuum provides a framework for evaluating the many levels of energy that people with long-term fatigue are dealing with at any point in time. For most of us, we are in energy rationing, but you are most likely trending towards one end of the continuum or the other — towards low or high energy.

It's important to note that these points are based on your current energy levels, which you may find for all intents and purposes has become your new normal. This is not a comparison to the amount of energy you used to have, or indeed want to have!

You can use this is to build up an understanding of what your average week looks like. Taking this as a guide, you can then evaluate how much activity you can realistically take on over your week.

This becomes your guide, but anyone dealing with fatigue for long enough will also know that any one week can also fluctuate wildly. You may have days of extremely low energy when everything feels difficult, like moving through thick molasses! The next day you are back to energy rationing, finding you have more energy available to do what needs to be done.

Even after my seven years with fatigue, I'm still at the point of energy rationing. Most days I'm on the high end of the continuum, around a 6 or 7, and can trust that my energy will consistently allow me to work in the mornings. Some days I still wake up and think, *'Nope, not today. I'm back down to a 4!'*

As others have accurately described, it can be difficult to predict where you will be on your continuum each day. I've come to accept that these fluctuations are also part of my new normal — at least for now.

Evaluating where you sit on average on your energy continuum is a good starting point. You can use this understanding to define the full set of rules, even your new normal, that needs to apply to best manage your current energy levels. Understanding these rules and how they apply to your situation sets the foundation for how you will then put the measures in place to live within your limits.

The following 'rules' — or principles that I decided I would need to live by — can be used to determine *your* new normal as well.

- Rule 1 — Your energy is now finite
- Rule 2 — You have an energy allowance
- Rule 3 — Your battery needs more frequent recharging
- Rule 4 — You need to make energy choices

What new set of rules are you living by? Let's break down each one in more detail to better define what your new normal has become.

Rule 1 — Your energy is now finite.

Energy is a resource often taken for granted. For someone with long-term fatigue, accounting for changes in fatigue and energy levels, the reality is you will end up with a fraction of the overall energy you are used to having. You may even start to view energy as your most precious resource!

Finite energy usually translates to less usable time during your day. For an average (non-fatigued) person, allocating 8 hours for sleep, you will have about 16 usable hours left for what you need to do. This is usually activities like caring, working, resting, relaxing, socialising, errands, projects, hobbies, household chores like cooking, cleaning, as well as the myriad of other responsibilities that we all hold.

With fatigue, usable hours can be low and completing activities often requires significant periods of rest in between. You will also most likely have times during the day that you are most active and able to maximise your usable hours. There will be other times when your energy plummets.

Finite energy and lowered usable hours usually significantly affect your ability to work full-time, or even maintain part-time hours. For some, work is the last to be cut back or given away completely out of necessity. This can mean other aspects of life are cut first, such as social occasions or health and wellness activities like cooking and exercise. For others, work is the first thing to go as their body cannot sustain the load.

In the beginning, you may try to keep up with the previous version of yourself, or at least keep up with the responsibilities present in your life. This ignores the fact that your energy has declined, and your growing need to plan activity around this reality. Decreasing amounts of usable hours becomes unavoidable, usually dictated by what your body will no longer allow you to do.

Eventually, an acceptance grows that you are now working with finite energy. Over time, your knowledge will build, understanding the fluctuations in your energy overall and defining how to manage your finite energy each day.

Once you understand and accept this big-picture concept of finite energy, you can take steps to quantify your energy allowance and better explain this concept for both you and others.

Rule 2 — You have an energy allowance.

The next of my rules or principles is about converting the intangible and vague notion of finite energy and your energy envelope into something that you can more readily understand and communicate.

You have a certain amount of energy to 'spend' in your day, which is your energy allowance. I outline two methods of quantifying this allowance that each communicate in different ways. You can choose the method that best resonates with you or use both.

- Method 1 — Spoon theory
- Method 2 — Energy 'units'

We'll start with spoon theory — an effective way of quantifying the energy cost of activities you choose to do within your day.

Method 1 — Spoon theory

Spoon theory is a fantastic metaphor that is widely helping people with chronic conditions manage their energy and plan their days. As an added side benefit, it is also a great tool for helping the people around you understand the concept of finite energy and how serious long-term fatigue can be.

Spoon theory[21] was created by Christine Miserandino who has lupus. She was eating dinner with a friend who asked her what it was like to live with her condition. Christine grabbed as many spoons as she could find and allocated each spoon one unit of energy.

With long-term fatigue, you don't have unlimited energy, or in this example, unlimited spoons. Instead, you might wake up and only have a few spoons' worth of energy to get you through the day. It then comes down to the choices you make on how to use this finite amount of energy available.

If you break down every task that your day holds, you can start to see how your energy is allocated.

- **Tasks can be simple** — such as getting out of bed, getting dressed, cleaning up after a meal, changing outfits. The 'cost' is only 1 spoon.
- **Tasks can also be more complex** — such as getting yourself to work, attending a health or medical appointment, spending time socialising. The 'cost' is 2 or more spoons.

---

21 You can read Christine Miserandino's full blog post explaining spoon theory here — butyoudontlooksick.com/articles/written-by-christine/the-spoon-theory

In a day, you might take on the following activities:

Activity	Spoons (energy cost)
1. Get up	1
2. Shower / wash up	2
3. Get dressed	1
4. Make and eat meal	2
5. Clean up kitchen after meal	1
6. Travel to health appointment	3
7. Attend health appointment	4
8. Travel home	3
9. Make and eat meal	2
10. Clean up kitchen after meal	1
11. Change into pyjamas	1
TOTAL	21

Table 3 — Activity and Spoons (Energy Cost)

Using Miserandino's spoon theory, you can allocate spoons or the energy cost, to each of the activities. The simple tasks like getting up and getting dressed might be 1 spoon. The larger tasks such as travelling and attending your appointment might take up a lot more energy. In this case, you can see the spoon cost of travelling to and from and attending a health appointment is a total of 10 spoons (activities 6 + 7 + 8).

Depending on where you are on the energy continuum, you will wake up with a certain number of spoons to use for the day.

If you only have 10 spoons' worth of energy to use, you have already used your allocation before you even attend your appointment! No wonder you are exhausted!

Anything you are doing that day from the appointment onwards is borrowing energy from the next day. This is where our boom-and-bust PEM cycle comes into play.

Dealing with long-term fatigue, the number of spoons or energy you have on any one day will vary, but you can start to see why getting out of bed and doing the basics are just so draining on your worst days. On your better days, you might have more than 21 spoons of energy, making all the activity listed in the table and more entirely possible.

Using this information, you can make an assessment each morning as to how many spoons you are likely to have for the day and plan accordingly.

Spoon theory is an excellent way of visually communicating the effects of finite energy, particularly describing it to the people around you for their own better understanding of your condition. Welcome to the 'spoonies' club!

Method 2 — Energy 'units'

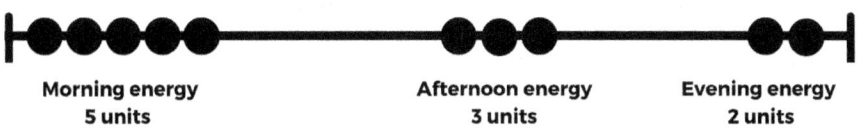

Figure 8 — Energy Units

Not everyone likes spoons! In the past before I'd even heard of spoons, I used a similar analogy by numbering my energy 'units'.

I like the number 10 and used to explain that I only have 10 units of energy for the whole day. Each activity costs me units and when I run out, I'm out of energy for the day. I then need a substantial rest period, or to retire entirely until I'm recharged again.

My day is also broken up with regular rest periods between activities and/or at certain times of the day.

An example:

- **Morning energy** — I feel the best in the mornings so I do some activity that adds up to 5 units. I then rest and recover.
- **Afternoon energy** — Around 3pm, I take my dog for a short walk, which requires a lot of energy, 3 units. I then rest and recover.
- **Evening energy** — I have enough energy to cook dinner and engage with my family, adding up to 2 units. After this, I retire to bed.

This might be a normal energy profile for my day. Your energy profile will vary. You can slide those energy units along the line in any formation you like!

On those bad days, you might only have 5 units of energy for the whole day. Or 2 units. You might use all your energy in the morning and get no afternoon or evening energy at all. Many combinations are possible.

The amount is not as important as the concept of limited energy that can be 'spent'. The variable amount of energy you have in any one day accounts for your current level of what is 'normal' and where you fall on the energy continuum.

As with your daily spoon allowance, each morning you can assess how you're tracking with your energy units and use this to plan your day.

Whatever method or metaphor works best for you, both are excellent ways of being able to understand your energy allowance and how much energy you have to 'spend' for the day. With this in place, you can then start to plan your rest and recharge periods.

Rule 3 — Your battery needs more frequent recharging.

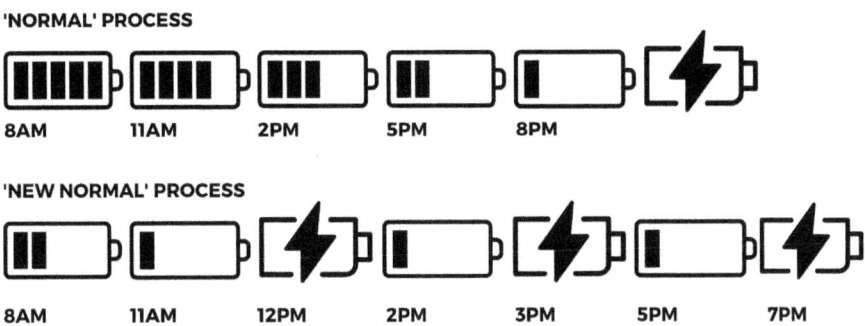

Figure 9 — Your Energy Battery

We saw that the energy continuum is about the amount of charge you have in your energy battery. Consider your body is a battery and your energy is the charge. In the past, you have most likely started your day waking up with a full battery. This battery charge will then last you through the day, until you go to sleep at night and recharge. You might experience dips during the day and need certain activities (or cups of coffee) to give you a boost, but for the most part you are able to get through to the evening.

With long-term fatigue, it can be that your battery is faulty and needs more frequent charging throughout the day! Your new normal is waking up without a full charge. Not only this, but your recharging dock can also be extremely slow!

The outcome is you start the day with only 50% charge (or 20% charge, or 10%). You then run low quite quickly and rely on your rest periods to boost your battery. Each rest period might only give you a 10% boost, so you need to keep recharging regularly throughout the day just to get through.

You retire at night with a low or flat battery and the whole process starts again!

Understanding your recharging requirements will help you schedule your rest and recharge sessions throughout the day. This may be downtime, sensory deprivation, sleep or some other activity like meditation or mindfulness.

Once you understand what rest and recharge you need during your day, it can become a process of making choices around what activities you choose to do around these rest periods with the amount of energy you have for the day.

Rule 4 — You need to make energy choices.

The rules until now have been around understanding your new limitations and requirements within your daily schedule. This is where you can start to take action.

Concepts like spoon theory and understanding your energy allowance demonstrate the heartbreaking choices we make every day around our energy usage. Accounting for your finite energy, you will eventually land on the fact that you can no longer squeeze the same amount of activity into your day as you once did. This is when, at their heart, your days become about making choices, such as how much you can push, when to rest and the best use of your energy for that day.

An analogy you may have come across is that of a rubber band. If you can imagine your energy choices you make are pulling your band tight, ideally leading to your rubber band having just enough tension to take form. Not enough tension on your band and it's too loose to function properly, but pull it too far and it snaps or rebounds back, slapping you in the face! In the same way, you are looking to find the balance of enough activity that provides benefit, but not so much that it rebounds and results in those negative consequences.

The choices you make in keeping your rubber band taut will be influenced by where you are on your energy continuum. You will most likely experience fluctuations in energy levels, based on your symptom triggers and the amount of PEM you experience. These energy fluctuations, how many usable hours you have in your day, what type of rest and recharge you need — all these factors will impact what choices you can make.

Often our choices are around planning a week in advance to even out the energy expenditure. It can become a trade-off. It might be that you have an event to attend or a task you need to finish and use more energy than you know is good for you. With long-term fatigue, you are not able to will more energy into your day. Rather the choice becomes whether you will borrow energy from the days to come, knowing that you are likely going to face the PEM consequences. Sometimes it's worth it; sometimes you'll live to regret it!

These days, I manage the tautness of my rubber band on a daily, weekly and monthly basis. When scheduling activities, taking on new projects and managing my day-to-day diary, I am constantly assessing my physical, mental and emotional load. I schedule in my rest periods first and build my schedule around those, knowing energy fluctuations will mean I might need more rest on some days and have more energy on others.

Some of the choices you make are not a fair choice or a kind choice, but they are a choice nonetheless. Depending on how much your energy fluctuates, it can be extremely difficult to estimate what your daily experience is going to be, varying from higher energy one day and crashing the next. This makes it difficult to make plans and stick to them or take on steady employment knowing you might experience a crash and not be able to fulfil your responsibilities.

Understanding these patterns goes a long way to helping you make those choices around the level of activity available to you and how you want to structure your week in order to keep your rubber band as taut as possible. More than ever, I'm now aware of the constant choices I'm making around the use of my energy — focusing on making informed choices that are in my own best interests.

Most of all, I've established a routine of activity that allows me to achieve my best within a new normal pace of life.

Using the rules to define your new normal

These rules represent your first step — understanding the rules and how they apply to your situation, and eventually defining your new normal. This sets the foundation for how you will then put the measures in place to live within your limits.

This alone can be a dramatic change of thinking. Before you have fully understood and adapted to the new set of rules being imposed, you might still be trying to squeeze the same amount of activity into your day. I and so many people I've spoken to are often still trying to keep up with the previous version of ourselves, or at least keep up with the responsibilities present in our life.

This might be a result of external pressure felt from others. More often, it's an internal pressure, holding onto a previous identity that is telling us what is possible, rather than facing the physical reality that our body is tired and requires new choices. We completely ignore the fact that we only have a certain amount of spoons' worth of energy to spend, or only 10 energy units that can be used over certain times of the day, and we're dealing with a faulty battery that barely keeps its charge!

This chapter has been all about moving the needle on your perspective of energy, starting to embrace the fact that you indeed have finite energy, an ever-moving energy envelope and you might even learn to define a new normal. This won't necessarily be permanent, but it is your physical reality

— at least for now. The quicker you can get your head around what are your energy limits, the quicker you can then start to change the pace of your life to one that supports you and puts you on a better path to healing.

The next chapter shows you the way to establish a routine of activity that works for your energy levels, aptly called pacing. Pacing is a hugely important concept in managing long-term fatigue, maybe even *the* most effective way of managing your current energy situation.

Putting it into practice

Take a moment to consider the 'rules' for managing your finite energy.

1. Where are you on the energy continuum currently and which way are you trending?

Rule 1 — Your energy is now finite.

2. How many usable hours do you have in your day (accounting for energy fluctuations)?
3. Are you trying to do an appropriate amount of activity for the usable hours you have available? If not, what do you need to manage?

Rule 2 — You have an energy allowance.

4. Using spoon theory or energy 'units', how many spoons or units' worth of energy do you have in an average day and how do you typically allocate them?
5. If you were to divide your energy into 10 equal units for an average day, how would you distribute them across morning, afternoon and evening?

Rule 3 — Your battery needs more frequent recharging.

6. What rest period is required after completing activity?
7. What type of activities allow you to rest and recharge, such as sleeping, sensory deprivation, sitting quietly, meditating etc.?

Rule 4 — You need to make energy choices.

8. What are some of the choices you've had to make to date based on your energy fluctuations?
9. What choices have you not yet made and see coming up in your future around your use of energy?

Chapter 5

Learning to Love Pacing

Sandy, a 53-year-old physiotherapist from Cork in Ireland, recalls having a particularly bad day managing her fatigue. She'd done everything right after resting, hydrating, gentle stretching and taking supplements. On this day, she had to be at work by 9am, but after getting up and trying to take a shower she felt terrible — shaky, unrefreshed, heart racing and very emotional.

She was frustrated and not sure what else she could have done. What hurt possibly the most was the thought of impacting her work colleagues (again) as she was clearly not able to work that day.

On reflection, Sandy could see that she had tried to return to part-time work too quickly after being diagnosed with long-COVID. She was able to discuss with her workplace occupational therapist a more staggered approach to recommencing work activity. They integrated pacing concepts of taking more regular rest breaks throughout her days and building up her hours slowly. Relaxation at home between shifts also became her priority.

With these changes, Sandy started improving. At times, progress felt painstakingly slow, but she learnt to recognise it as progress nonetheless and the way her new normal had to be — for the time being at least.

You might recall my lack of skills in managing energy when first diagnosed with chronic fatigue syndrome and the crash course I took in energy management while in the throes of managing fatigue. I was really affected by this new set of rules that was suddenly thrust upon me.

These rules dictated my life — I had very little energy to use in the day and would be absolutely slammed for days to come if I did too much. There were too many days that I accidently crossed the invisible line of activity that my body allowed, and my rubber band rebounded swiftly to slap me across the face!

My managing energy quick-start program relied heavily on a concept I now know as pacing, arguably *the* best treatment protocol we have for the management of long-term fatigue. At the start, I did not love pacing — not at all! Our relationship was pure resentment on my behalf. Yet over time, I've come to embrace it as a more sustainable way to run my life. I've now also recognised the effectiveness of pacing for managing all our lives, providing great benefit beyond just the confines of fatigue.

What is pacing?

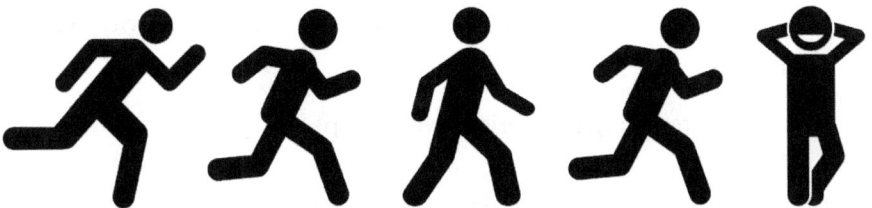

Figure 10 — Pacing in Action

To give you an analogy, imagine you are running a race. The whistle blows and you take off full speed, jostling for position. You keep this pace up for a while, but realise you are getting tired and out of breath. You slow down to a comfortable jog, focusing on breathing deeply and taking regular steps. When you come to hills you slow down even further. You rest at the water stops. You speed up at certain points when you feel an energy burst, but make sure you slow down to your comfortable jog when the energy fades.

This is an example of pacing — finding a comfortable rhythm that allows you to last the distance.

With long-term fatigue, pacing is about establishing a routine of activity that works to your energy levels.

On any one day…

- You start with your regular activity (whistle blows, you begin the race).
- You do an activity that is mentally draining for 15 minutes (slowing down to a comfortable jog).
- You take a restoring rest period (water stop).
- You feel fatigue rising and do your next activity mindfully (walking, not jogging, up the hill).

- You take a restoring rest period (water stop).
- You feel your energy rising and do a short physical activity (energy burst).
- You take a restoring rest period (water stop).

Just like the race, running your day using pacing is about finding a rhythm that is comfortable and achievable.

Pacing might seem like a simple concept, but can be extremely difficult to implement. It is basically the practical application of putting your new set of rules into action. The overall goal is to manage your energy and activity levels to avoid overexertion and worsen your fatigue symptoms. There is a balance here — between doing the activity you want to do in your day, building rest in between activities and avoiding the dreaded boom-and-bust cycle.

I was a bit of slow learner when it came to pacing, most likely not aided by my gung-ho personality and mind that always seems to be on! It took me a long time to wrap my head around the concept that I would not be able to do it all — work, social, learning, adventures, the list went on.

I needed to drop most of what I did for a while as I got used to a new normal level of energy. The PEM I experienced as I got used to this new normal was excruciating, confining me to bed for days at a time.

Pacing eventually became an automatic part of my mindset. Instinctively, I knew I needed to balance my energy throughout the week. If I did something strenuous one day, I started to 'budget' for rest in the days that followed. Somewhere along the line, most likely when reaching my new normal, my attitude towards pacing changed from resentment to acceptance. This is the level of activity I am allowed — at least for now.

Pacing incorporates adequate rest and recharge

Remember Rule 3 — at its heart, pacing builds those rest and recharge periods into your day. Rest involves many options, including sleep, sensory deprivation, listening to music or podcasts, watching TV, reading, practicing self-care activities such as meditation, stretching or gentle exercise to help promote relaxation. Maybe what works for you is just doing nothing. There is no set activity for rest — it depends entirely on you.

Some days you might need minimal rest periods; others you need a lot. For me, some of my days became one big rest period — the day never really got started! And that's okay. I learnt to listen to what my body needed.

Gradually, you're learning to treat these rest breaks like the precious time they are. Rest and recharge help prevent further fatigue and give you the boost of energy needed so you can do the activities that mean the most to you. When you start feeling fatigued, it's usually a sign to take a break or adjust your pace to conserve that precious energy.

Have you learnt to love pacing yet?

If you have been living with long-term fatigue for a while, you're most likely an expert at pacing, even if you don't recognise it as such. If you're not quite an expert yet, it could be something to aspire to!

Human nature can be to fight it at the beginning. For some of us, the decision is made for you, and you'll have no choice but to learn to pace yourself as part of your experience. For others, it can be that you try to soldier on, doing all that you need to do. At some point you'll inevitably realise that you just can't do it all and need to be kinder to yourself.

This often involves a fight between the mind and the body — we want to continue living life as we always have, but our body has other ideas!

I know the bitter disappointment of not being able to attend a long-awaited event as you are just too fatigued that day. Or like Sandy in the opening snapshot of this chapter, the angst at feeling like you are letting people down when you cannot complete a work task or attend work at all due to your fatigue.

I accept that these feelings are deeply uncomfortable, but when the trade-off becomes severe PEM or even more angst at time off work, then you know you are making choices for yourself that are in your own best interest. You are learning to love pacing for the relief it can provide to your fatigue.

How do you incorporate pacing into your lifestyle?

The overall goal of pacing is about managing the energy you have in a day to achieve what you need while minimising the resulting PEM. A more subtle part of the equation is application of Rule 1, coming to a point of acceptance that you can't do it all — at least not for now.

There are many paths to implementing pacing. Here are just some of the ways that others have gone about it.

1. **Breaking tasks into manageable chunks,** such as starting a task in the morning, having a break, then finishing it in the afternoon or the next day.
2. **Taking regular breaks** when needed to avoid pushing yourself too hard. This involves listening to your body and responding when you start feeling fatigued or experiencing symptoms.
3. **Adjusting the pace and intensity** of the activity based on how it feels and how much energy you have in that day.
4. **Scheduling only one significant activity in a day,** such as a work task, a social occasion or household chores like groceries and cooking.

5. **Saying 'no' when required with comfort and ease,** knowing how much activity you can handle over a day or week, prioritising what is most important to you and giving yourself permission to decline invitations with grace.

6. **Using tools such as timers, alarms or activity trackers** to help manage time and energy. An example is the Pomodoro Technique, which uses 25-minute stretches of focus time, followed by 5-minute rest intervals or sometimes a longer break.

7. **Prioritising activities based on the energy levels** you feel on the day and making sure the most important tasks are completed first.

8. **Gradually increasing activity levels over time** to build your stamina.

9. **Email strategies** such as using your autoresponder or out-of-office functionality to help manage expectations of when you will reply.

10. **Professional support** such as mentoring or coaching to improve your pacing skills, identify where your mindset might be holding you back or causing distress, and ultimately setting you up for pacing success.

While pacing becomes crucial in the ongoing management of fatigue, it's also useful to consider its benefit in our hectic and often exhausting modern lives. Many of these strategies have proven to be of use more widely, regardless of whether you have a fatigue condition or not.

Implementing pacing strategies

Implementing pacing is often about trial and error. Unfortunately, it is never an exact science, and you might need to try out some of these strategies to find what works best for you.

You've seen there are frequent fluctuations in your energy levels, depending on where you are on the energy continuum. Pacing might never be something you can 100% get right, but you can use it to respond the best you can to how you are feeling on the day.

Here's what I've noticed about pacing and how you can define it for yourself.

Pacing is:

- **Prioritising** — Using your energy for the things that matter most and what needs to be done first, knowing you may not get to the items lower on the list.

- **Accepting the consequences** — Sometimes pushing yourself harder than advised when you absolutely have to or want to do certain activities. You do this knowing there will likely be consequences and you need to schedule your recovery time.

- **Tuning in** — Listening to your body, understanding what you are capable of on any one day and adjusting accordingly.

- **Scheduling rest** — Building in regular rest and recovery periods throughout your days and across your week.

- **Managing those around you** — Communicating clearly and setting good boundaries to create reasonable expectations and maintain good relationships.

The goal is for you to become a pacing expert and establish a routine of activity that works for your situation. This involves getting good at listening to your body and adjusting your activity and schedule as needed. When you realise the benefits pacing provides for managing fatigue, that is when your love of pacing will truly start to kick in!

Pacing is the key to (eventual) improvement in symptoms and getting your life back to a regular routine, adapting to your new normal. Cultivating a positive and healing mindset around all these changes will be our next area of focus.

Putting it into practice

Take a moment to review how you incorporate pacing into your day.

1. Do you have your pacing right at the moment?
2. Do you have a comfortable rhythm throughout your day?
3. Do you have adequate rest and recovery periods?
4. What strategies do you use to implement pacing into your lifestyle?
5. What 'rules' do you follow when implementing pacing?
6. Do those around you understand and help accommodate your pacing requirements?
7. What else do you need to consider in your quest of learning to love pacing?

Physical Summary

- Long-term fatigue conditions, such as ME/CFS, fibromyalgia and long-COVID, can be complex, largely hidden conditions where people face similar challenges. They are often not well-understood — by yourself, those around you or the medical community.

- Symptoms of these conditions can be vague and varied. Apart from fatigue, symptoms include brain fog, body aches, gastrointestinal issues, dizziness, sleep issues, mood impacts, PEM and POTS.

- PEM is central to diagnosis for any long-term fatigue condition. It is the after-effects from physical, mental and emotional exertion. PEM is frequently accompanied by boom-and-bust cycles.

- Managing your finite energy starts with understanding your current energy envelope, or the amount of energy you have available each day, using your energy continuum. This may change daily.

- Managing your energy comes down to a set of principles, or 'rules', eventually used to understand and define your new normal.

  Rule 1 — Your energy is now finite.
  Rule 2 — You have an energy allowance.
  Rule 3 — Your battery needs more frequent recharging.
  Rule 4 — You need to make energy choices.

- Pacing is about establishing a routine of activity that works to your energy levels. Incorporating pacing into your lifestyle involves taking adequate rest breaks and prioritising what is most important for you to achieve.

- Reaching your new normal comes with a level of peace and acceptance — focusing your valuable energy on the things that matter most and building a sustainable pace of life.

Emotional Reality...
Riding the Rollercoaster

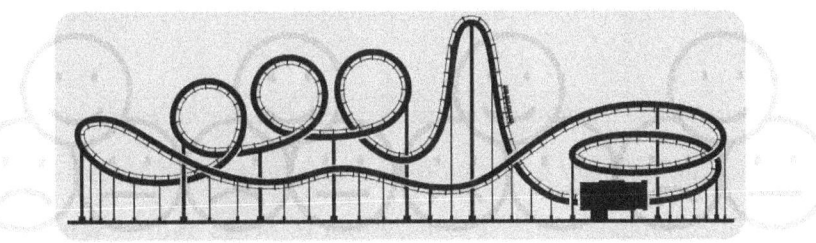

I changed the rules. I was in a loving, committed relationship of five years when disaster struck in the form of my exhaustion. Seemingly overnight, I went from being communicative, loving and giving to feeling grouchy, introverted and sad. I wanted to come out of my room, but I felt completely depleted — like I had nothing left to give. My room became my sanctuary and the only place I felt safe. I could feel the change and my partner pulling away, but felt powerless to do anything about it. Honestly, just getting through each day was hard enough already.

Living with long-term fatigue can have a significant impact on your emotional wellbeing. We've already covered a lot of ground as to why this might be the case.

To recap:

- It's a **hidden condition,** notoriously difficult to understand by everyone around you (including yourself!).
- You will most likely experience a **multitude of different symptoms**.
- You seemingly cross **an invisible line** in activity levels and are hit hard with PEM.
- It brings with it a **new set of rules** for managing your energy.
- You're probably not sure what to **expect from yourself** on any one day.
- You'll continually **traverse a marathon of peaks and troughs** as you chase improvement and recovery.

There's a lot to work with here!

Before we dive into this important section, as this book only contains general advice, please seek your own individualised medical and mental health care where appropriate. If you need help or someone to talk to, if this material is triggering, and especially if you have thoughts of self-harm, seek support and choose an option that's right for you. For some, it will be family and friends. There are also professional support sources such as a counsellor, psychologist, or psychiatrist. Most often, it will be a combination of these support options[22].

---

[22] Options also include support lines - you can reach Lifeline on 13 11 14 in Australia, or 0808 808 8000 in the UK, and the Suicide and Crisis Lifeline on 988 in the USA. Other countries' support lines can be found here: en.wikipedia.org/wiki/List_of_suicide_crisis_lines

You've probably come to realise that the physical symptoms sound awful (and they are), but it can be the psychological impact that hurts the most. 'Long-term' means it will affect you day after day, month after month. For some, it's even year after year. It can be relentless and often hits people in their prime years — at times cutting down promising careers and ruining lives in extreme cases.

I've had many dark thoughts over the years, an experience commonly echoed by others with long-term fatigue. When you suffer a relentless condition that continually compromises your ability to do the things you once could, it's easy to fall into patterns of despair.

Despairing thoughts I've entertained over the years include:

- Ever being productive again — *'Will I ever be able to work/travel/enjoy life in the same way again?'*
- Having fulfilling friendships and a partner — *'Who would want me now?'*
- Being worthy of living — *'What use am I to anyone?'*

These thoughts are a one-way street to misery or worse, and they require a 'fight' to manage them. However, this fight requires energy and is energetically 'expensive', as well as being difficult to command when you are fatigued.

Let me start by validating these feelings. It can be hard. It's heavy, silent, exhausting…not just taxing on your physical energy, but also on your very life-force, your get-up-and-go. It doesn't seem fair, and it isn't. Most likely those around you cannot easily understand, so it can also be lonely.

These are all valid emotions that no doubt anyone battling long-term fatigue has experienced at some point in time. You are definitely not alone in this.

You will most likely have good and bad days. At times, it might seem more bad than good. On these days, it can be easy to think you'll never be any different and that things will never change. You might feel lost in your condition. You don't recognise the person looking back at you in the mirror. You feel like you have lost who you once were, maybe even forever.

Like anything in life, it's how we approach these situations that make a difference. There are also good times and positive stories that come out of these experiences. Frequently, new layers of support are established. Lessons are learnt around supportive boundaries, good lifestyle practices and being able to speak out where you once could not.

In your marathon event, there are no quick fixes. Instead, you'll find it takes time. You need space. Changes in lifestyle and beliefs. New habits. New pathways and ways of thinking. Most of all, you need courage to take it on, patience when it seems impossible and perseverance to get you through.

These qualities I'm describing are strengths. You might be more focused on the weakness you feel in your body and mind. We often judge ourselves harshly in these circumstances. However, for those of us navigating a long-term condition like fatigue, we're demonstrating courage, patience and perseverance in action.

Do these seem like qualities of a weak person to you?
How much stronger would you feel after getting through such a period? It's often life-defining, and it can even be viewed as a gift. A gift you neither asked for nor even wanted, but a gift nonetheless!

This section will help you build that strong, resilient, healing mindset required to navigate your marathon journey. It will allow you to grieve the loss of the person you once were, adapting to the new normal physical and lifestyle limitations you are experiencing. It will help you develop the mindset you need to not only manage your day-to-day experiences, but also to support the growth you are so capable of achieving.

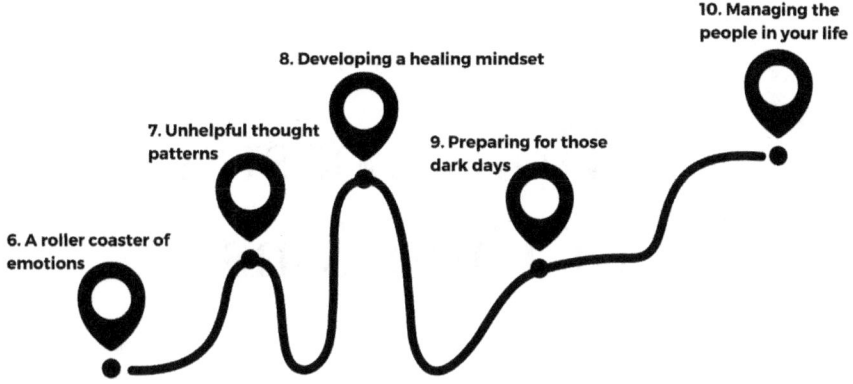

Figure 11 — Emotional Reality Chapter Roadmap

- Chapter 6 is about managing the rollercoaster of emotions that accompany this condition — the complex mix of energy and hope along with the inevitable slides into pits of despair.

- Chapters 7 and 8 identify the unhelpful thinking patterns you might be entertaining and show you what's needed to train your mind in order to be able to handle any challenge in life.

- Chapters 9 and 10 look at your ability to cope with even the darkest days and to build the team of navigation partners you need for a better future.

This is your emotional reality: how you ride the waves of emotions and tap into a mindset that is about growth and support. Your marathon journey will most likely not be entirely without its dark days, but this section will show you the tools to eventually emerge triumphantly into the light.

Chapter 6
A Rollercoaster of Emotions

Kimi was 42, working as an HR manager in a high-stress corporate environment when she finally had to admit something was very wrong. She was crying a lot — before work, at lunchtime, on the way home from work and in the evenings. Crying can be cathartic and a release, but this much outpouring was hard to take both physically and mentally. It was also difficult to hide, and after having such a long and successful career, Kimi really didn't want people knowing how bad her emotional state had become.

Strangely, her crying alternated with bouts of extreme anger. It was beyond infuriation; she was absolutely outraged at the smallest things such as slow-walking people, waiting more than a minute for her coffee order to be made, or perceived slights in the workplace such as someone not holding the elevator door for her! How could people be so inconsiderate?

Kimi had been denying what she'd been feeling for a long time. The mind-numbing fatigue was her constant companion — she needed to dramatically scale back her daily routine and seek help. She resisted for so long due to feelings of guilt and shame and not wanting to let anyone down. Eventually, her body made the choice for her, and she was forced to drop down to part-time work, which if she was honest, was a welcome relief.

Anyone enduring a long-term condition will most likely experience a rollercoaster of emotions, fatigue being no exception. There are several factors when dealing with fatigue that can add to your load and result in emotional difficulty:

- **It's a marathon** — Long-term fatigue can be a marathon event, often lasting years. This adds difficulty not only for the person dealing with fatigue, but for those around them to remain patient and understanding, at times picking up the slack.

- **There's a lack of predictability** — Each day brings different energy levels. As you ride the rollercoaster of peaks and troughs, it can be difficult to predict what is going to be possible. Some days are good; some you can barely get out of bed.

- **Peaks are difficult to come by and often followed by troughs** — The pattern of improvement and recovery is not linear. Sometimes it seems like it's two steps forward, one step (or even three steps) back! Feeling improvement in your energy (your peaks) is joyous, but it can make the feeling of the next loss of momentum or dip in energy (your troughs) difficult to accept.

- **Progress is out of your control** — As humans, we are drawn to certainty and a sense of 'fairness'. Fatigue is a condition where patterns of improvement can seem largely out of your control, messing with this sense of fair play. This can feel devastating when you put so much effort into improving your energy, only to regress on certain days, seemingly without reason.

- **Symptoms are vague and difficult to explain** — Understanding the assortment of symptoms that commonly accompany long-term fatigue can take a long time. The challenge then becomes trying to explain your experience to the people around you in a way that they can understand, and that you feel seen and heard.
- **The way forward is unclear** — There is no one treatment protocol nor single set of recommendations that will help all people. It becomes hit or miss finding helpful practitioners and treatments that make a difference to your fatigue symptoms.

Considering the above, it is no surprise people with long-term fatigue suffer through this emotional rollercoaster. You can be forgiven for being fed up and frustrated with the whole process.

This rollercoaster is actually a normal part of the human experience and can be explained through a model known as the grief cycle.

The grief cycle explains how we process our emotions.

Elisabeth Kübler-Ross was a Swiss-American psychiatrist who developed a model around the cycle of human emotional states, referred to as the grief cycle. Through her work with terminally ill patients, Kübler-Ross identified a cycle of five stages of grief her patients commonly went through as they traversed their various illnesses.

In her book *On Death and Dying*[23], Kübler-Ross outlines these five stages of grief as follows:

1. **Denial** — Trying to avoid the inevitable. *'It's not true.'*
2. **Anger** — Frustrated outpouring of bottled-up emotion. *'It's not fair.'*
3. **Bargaining** — Offering deals as a method of seeking a way out. *'I'll do anything.'*
4. **Depression** — Downward swing as you realise the inevitable. *'What's the point?'*
5. **Acceptance** — A way forward, adjusting to a new reality. *'I can't change it.'*

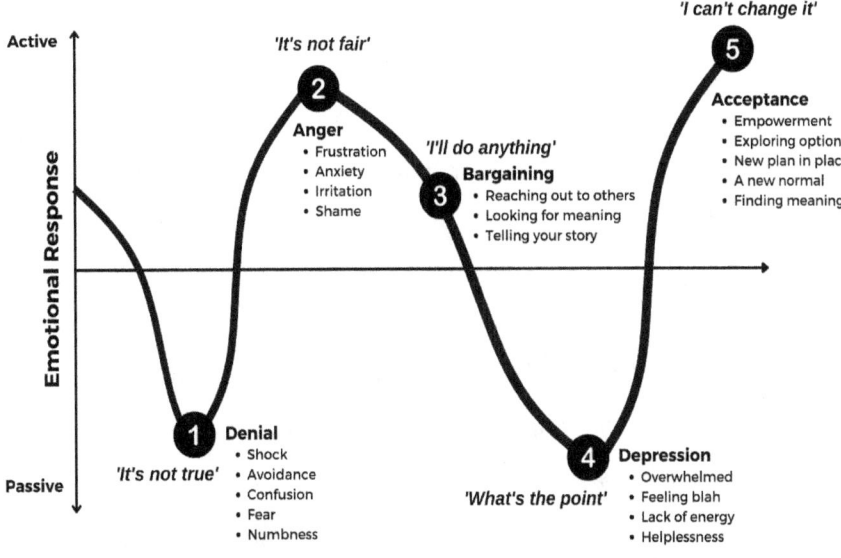

Figure 12 — Kubler Ross Grief Cycle

---

23 Reference: Elisabeth Kübler-Ross, On Death and Dying, Macmillan, NY, 1969

In the ensuing years, it's been recognised that this cycle is not just applicable for grief, but also useful for understanding the emotional rollercoaster travelled within a variety of other situations. Examples of these situations include: processing bad news, navigating big life changes and dealing with long-term conditions such as fatigue.

Our emotional cycle with fatigue

This model is fantastic for understanding the emotional cycle we navigate with long-term fatigue. As part of the rollercoaster of emotions, you will have your ups (joy, love, hope, elation, optimism etc). However, what goes up also comes down, and you will also be travelling those stages of grief as part of the process. Let's see how the grief cycle plays out in reality:

- **Denial** — *'I'm so tired all the time, but I'm just going to keep on doing the same activities as I've always done — I have to work after all.'*
- **Anger** — *'I'm finding it so frustrating that I can't do even the basics or get any straight answers from the medical system. I've been lashing out at those around me.'*
- **Bargaining** — *'I'll tell you what — if this weakness will just leave my body, then starting tomorrow I'll make the most of this new opportunity.'*
- **Anger** — *'I've had a bad day and feel mad at everyone and everything!'*
- **Depression** — *'This is it! It's been weeks of feeling awful and I feel like I'm never going to rid my body of this weakness. I feel sad and alone.'*
- **Anger** — *'Why is this happening to me? It's so unfair.'*
- **Bargaining** — *'If I can just have a good few days for that wedding I want to go to, I'll take whatever happens after.'*
- **Denial** — *'I'm feeling better lately so it must be all over. Yippee! I'm healed.'*

- **Anger** — *'Not this again. Why am I so exhausted when I've done everything I possibly can?'*
- **Acceptance** — *'I've recited the serenity prayer so many times I'm starting to believe it! I accept I cannot change what's happening to me right now.'*
- **Bargaining** — *'Once I get through this week, everything should calm down and I promise not to take on more than I can handle next time.'*
- **Depression** — *'This is relentless. That doctor didn't help me at all. I'm too tired to even be angry about it. I just feel helpless.'*

And so on…

You might have noticed that you don't necessarily experience the stages of grief in a linear fashion or in a fixed order. More likely, you're jumping between the stages — moving from denial to anger, then to bargaining and maybe depression. You may have moments of acceptance when you feel at peace, only to be thrown back into anger with a bad day or an unhelpful encounter.

Do you find yourself jumping around the stages? If so, you're completely normal! Every person is unique and will create their own individual experience when dealing with long-term fatigue. There is no one right order or timeframe for navigating this cycle.

With that in mind, our emotional reality will most likely be a jumble of negative emotions directed towards our situation, something like this:

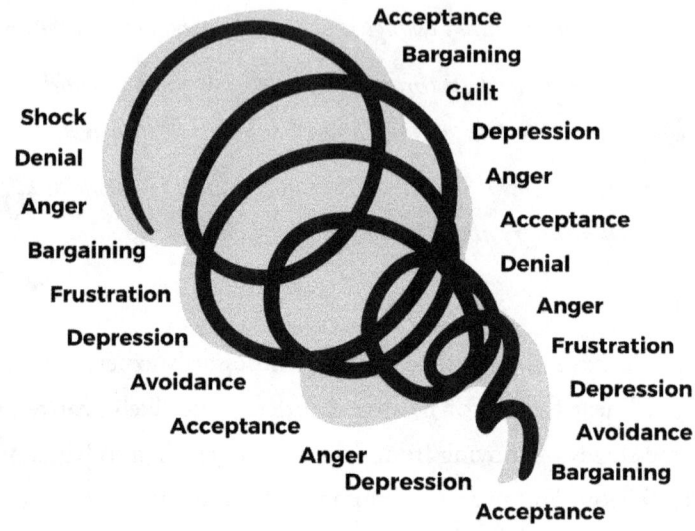

Figure 13 — Emotional Reality

You can see that you'll most likely flicker backwards and forwards between the stages of grief. Among all this flickering, one problem you might face is you get stuck in a certain stage.

- If you're stuck in **denial**, you're trying to not acknowledge your condition. You're still attempting to do all the things you once could, like keeping up a social life or attending work. Most likely you're exhausting yourself in the process.
- If you're stuck in **anger**, you may find yourself lashing out at the world, expending energy fighting what becomes a futile battle. This can alienate those around you.

- Being stuck in repeated **bargaining** might mean you are trying to find an acceptable deal that offers you a way out of your condition.

- You're stuck in **depression** when you're feeling deeply down, sad or lonely. Many of us will require medical assistance to manage these symptoms.

As we have explored, there is no timeline on how long you should be in each stage. It might take you a long while, years even, to come to grips and grieve your previous reality.

The most healing stage is **acceptance**. This stage can still see you having good and bad days, experiencing feelings such as sadness or pain. Bad days aside, in this stage you're at a level of peace with your condition and you have begun to adjust to a new reality.

Signs of reaching some level of acceptance include:

1. **Letting go** — You're not wasting energy fighting, feeling down about what's out of your control.

2. **Current reality** — You're being as proactive as possible, but acknowledging and able to vocalise your current reality — what you can and cannot do.

3. **Building a future** — You're starting to plan and make decisions for your future, considering what life will look like and how you will move forward.

4. **Meaning and purpose** — You're beginning to find new meaning and purpose with your life, even though your loss might still be felt. You might focus on positive memories and experiences.

As this is a cycle, you might feel acceptance for a while, but then find a bad day pushes you back into anger or depression. This is an unfortunate hallmark of dealing with long-term conditions — our tendency to continue cycling through the stages, especially on those bad days.

A marathon journey — overlaying your emotional cycles

If you think back to our marathon of improvement and recovery, you might be able to match up your emotional cycles with your physical reality. In particular, Stage 2 (messy middle) and Stage 3 (onwards and upwards) consist of a pattern of peaks and troughs.

- **In the physical peaks,** you're most likely to experience positive emotions, particularly hope, and be more inclined to embrace feelings of acceptance of your new normal and the limits this brings. For some, this can be a danger zone where we forget our limits or linger in denial that anything is wrong. When you feel more energetic for a while, you might end up overdoing things.
- **In the physical troughs,** you are most likely to feel negative emotions like anger or frustration. You may also feel down and depressed.

Our marathon journey involves these continual physical and emotional cycles. You might feel like you're improving and what an elated feeling that is! Then the next week, you crash back into the depths of frustration or depression.

This is the real marathon — finding ways to maintain your emotional peace of mind even on those darkest of days. The question becomes: how do we keep our hope and optimism alive throughout these patterns of peaks and troughs?

A sixth stage?

Subsequent to the development of Kübler-Ross's five stages of grief, her co-researcher David Kessler proposed the addition of a sixth stage, **meaning**[24]. This was one of the hallmarks for acceptance - you eventually start to find meaning or purpose arising from your grief and loss. This can be a truly transformative time in the process that allows you to grow from your experience.

In the words of Michael J. Fox, who has spent many years living with Parkinson's disease:

"Acceptance doesn't mean resignation. It means understanding that something is what it is and there's got to be a way through it."

It is through meaning that I have been able to channel the pain of my seven years with chronic fatigue syndrome into writing this book. My motivation stems from transforming my pain into developing a resource that provides valuable support, guidance and hope. In turn, this has given me a deep sense of meaning and purpose.

The next section begins your journey of proactively developing a mindset that best supports your emotional highs and lows, allowing you to be in the optimal frame of mind for healing. We begin by exploring some of the ways you might fail to help yourself — the unhelpful thought patterns that are so easy to slip into.

---

24 Reference: Kessler, David (2019), Finding Meaning: The sixth stage of grief, Sribner.

Putting it into practice

Spend a moment considering how you navigate the grief cycle in relation to your condition.

1. What behaviours do you find yourself exhibiting at each stage?

    1. Denial —
    2. Anger —
    3. Bargaining —
    4. Depression —
    5. Acceptance —

2. Do you have an emotional 'home', i.e. your go-to emotion? What is this emotion and how does it show up for you?
3. Are you (or have you ever been) stuck in any of the stages?
4. What do you think you can do to become unstuck?
5. If the sixth stage is meaning, how can you relate your condition to this?

Chapter 7
Unhelpful Thought Patterns

Margaret from Brighton in the UK was 68 when her levels of fatigue regressed to the point where she needed a wheelchair to get around. She found it torturous at first. Although it was a great relief physically, psychologically she suffered. She wondered if people thought she was a fraud because she still looked quite healthy.

This brought on feelings of guilt that she should force herself to walk. Living in a society that valued contribution, Margaret felt stuck — like she wasn't contributing. If she let it, this could become a perpetual cycle of guilt and pain.

Making light of situations and keeping her sense of humour alive was one of the strategies Margaret and her husband employed to make the darker days just that little bit brighter. Margaret's fun personality shone through as she learnt to embrace her new wheels, travelling at maximum speed when out in public. Based on her track record of reversing into shop displays and the occasional bumping of pedestrians, her husband eventually took out an insurance policy on her behalf, which provided great hilarity for them both!

Your mindset, or your frame of mind, is the set of perceptions and beliefs that shape how you make sense of the world and yourself. The mindset developed around your fatigue condition will never be all good or all bad. We tend to see things both positively and negatively, even simultaneously.

On certain days, you might find the positive prevails. You can see your fatigue as an opportunity and appreciate the lessons you've learnt in practicing self-care, rest and self-compassion. You operate with a growth mindset.

On other days, the negative takes over. You feel emotions such as guilt and shame. You might feel weak and start to resent what you cannot do. You might even resist or neglect the things you know will help, such as rest and self-care.

Some days are just a jumble of emotions, see-sawing between positive and negative mindsets!

This section will examine how your mindset is formed based on various inputs. In particular, you will think about how the negative elements develop, the unhelpful thought patterns. These often arise from your own biases or from the lack of empathy, judgements, negative comments or even disbelief that come your way.

These positive and negative influences on your mindset arise from a range of sources:

- **From family, friends, colleagues, neighbours** who can be helpful and encouraging towards your condition, but may also offer well-meaning but ultimately unhelpful advice, thoughtless commentary or unintentional pressure, which can have negative effects.

- **From medical practitioners** that are so helpful when you find a good source of support, helping you regain a sense of control and feel progress within your journey. On the other hand, an ill-informed practitioner will struggle to recognise your condition, let alone know what to do about it.
- **From ourselves** as you bring your own existing thought patterns and self-beliefs. How you viewed yourself in the past may have been tied to your external achievement. When you find this challenged, you can find your whole self-concept impacted in the form of self-judgements and negative inner dialogue, effectively sabotaging your healing journey.

Out of all these influences, you start from within. You have the power to manage how you perceive the commentary from elsewhere. Knowing this puts you in a place of strength to filter out the negativity or unhelpful comments from others. Sometimes doing this will be possible. Other times... easier said than done!

The struggle comes when you are not able to filter out thoughtless remarks and judgements. This makes your healing journey so much more difficult — trying to manage this becomes exhausting on top of an already exhausting situation. But perhaps the most impact comes from the self-sabotage that can be unleashed.

Self-sabotage[25] is the unhelpful programming that creeps into your mind, creating negative thought patterns or a negative mindset around your situation. Your thought patterns and mindset are predominantly formed in childhood. This patterning becomes ingrained over time, shaped by your experiences and interactions with others.

---

25 A comprehensive exploration of self-sabotage and all that it involves, including practical applications into work and life and extra resources, is available through positivepsychology.com.

A change in your physical state, such as that caused by fatigue, can severely impact how you view yourself, based on your own set of expectations. Margaret in the opening snapshot of this chapter demonstrated examples of this self-sabotage or unhelpful programming in action — experiencing guilt, feeling sad she couldn't contribute and worrying about how others might perceive her.

This self-sabotage can result in emotions like guilt or frustration, as well as judgements around your condition, particularly around what you can *no longer* do. You might start telling yourself stories such as that you are 'lazy', 'weak', 'a burden'… (insert your own word here). I found 'lazy' a particularly difficult judgement to shake over the years of managing my fatigue.

These judgements are often largely shaped by your family or your influences growing up and the beliefs they held. If you're not working hard or a 'go-getter', then you're lazy. If you're not able to help around the house, then you have nothing to contribute. Often, those in your inner circle will reinforce these old, unhelpful beliefs as that is what they know too.

Here's the problem… These judgements do not account for changes in circumstances such as illness or even just wanting a change in life. Your self-sabotage ends when you can make allowances for your condition and adapt to your new set of circumstances.

As we saw with Margaret, there are helpful approaches for overcoming these programming patterns and breaking out of the self-sabotage — such as using humour and embracing the way things are instead of sinking into that perpetual cycle of guilt and pain. In my own life, I found writing down my experiences in a diary an incredibly useful tool when I was struggling to see an end to my fatigue. It's allowed me to incorporate into this book those deepest of emotions experienced at the height of my fatigue in a very real way.

Later sections will explore how you too can overcome your own unhelpful programming and negative thought patterns, instead creating a more healing mindset. First, you need to identify the ways you're *not helping* yourself to heal and thrive, as well as what outside influences are reinforcing these self-sabotaging messages.

In the early days of my fatigue condition, I was misdiagnosed as just being stressed. While misdiagnosis is never great, the best thing that came out of this time was being prescribed a book by my doctor called *Change your Thinking*[26] by Dr Sarah Edelman. It turned out to be a great read, particularly the section that talks about faulty thinking.

'Faulty thinking' as a term is no longer in vogue, but it was used to describe unhelpful programming and negative thought patterns that overlay how you see the world. This is known as **cognitive distortion**, where your thought patterns are distorting your reality.

An article by Peter Grinspoon MD[27] aptly defines cognitive distortion as: '*…internal mental filters or biases that increase our misery, fuel our anxiety and make us feel bad about ourselves.*'

'Distortion' contributes to that unhelpful programming and causes emotional distress, resulting in a negative mindset around your condition. Ouch! Yes, that all rings very true.

I've found this negative mindset is most likely to occur when I'm at my weakest. It's easier to think positively about your future from a good headspace, but on those darkest days, things can start to look grim. Most likely, you see why it's so easy to fall into these unhelpful thought patterns when dealing with a long-term condition that is relentless — affecting you day-in, day-out.

---

26 Reference: Edelman, Sarah (2013), Change your thinking, ABC books.
27 Reference: Grinspoon, Peter (MD), How to recognize and tame your cognitive distortions, available at: www.health.harvard.edu

The following are the unhelpful thought patterns and examples that most often seem to affect myself and others with long-term fatigue.

- **Tyranny of the shoulds** — Believing things 'should' or 'must' be a certain way rather than simply having a preference. These become the rules or rigid beliefs you hold about yourself and the world around you.

    Examples where you 'should' or 'must': *I should be working and supporting myself. I should be getting better by now as it's been 12 months. I should always be positive even when I'm having a bad day. I should at least be able to run around the block, since I used to be able to do 5km. I must attend the family event no matter how bad I feel on the day.*

    Examples where you 'shouldn't' or 'mustn't': *I shouldn't have to rely on my family so much. I shouldn't need so much time to do this simple task. I shouldn't nap during the day or spend all day in bed. I shouldn't go a day without showering. I mustn't cancel on people or make plans I can't keep. I mustn't let anyone down.*

- **Catastrophising/awfulising** — Exaggerating the negative aspects of your life situations. You can have serious issues and a lot of negative aspects to work with when dealing with long-term fatigue, but this is about feeling distress that is worse than it needs to be.

    Examples: *Brain fog led me to forget to attend my hair appointment and now I can never go back there again. Getting sick means my life is ruined. If I feel this tired now, I'll never be able to function normally again.*

- **Black and white thinking** — Tendency to see things in a polarising way without acknowledging any middle ground, e.g. good or bad, right or wrong, success or failure, all or nothing. It ignores the fact that most things in life are about context and fall in between the extremes. Think shades of grey rather than black or white.

Examples: *This condition has completely ruined my future. My friends are either with me or against me, and if they do not ring me regularly, I am going to write them off. There is nothing good about my life right now. It is wrong that I have this condition. There's no point me even starting when I know I'm not going to be able to finish. Either this treatment works, or it was a complete waste of time.*

- **Overgeneralising** — Drawing negative conclusions based on limited evidence. You might find yourself saying things like 'always', 'never' and 'everybody', forgetting about times where you made gradual or slight improvement.

  Examples: *I'm never going to feel healthy again. I feel exhausted all the time. Everybody at work is out to get me. What use am I if I'm not achieving anything worthwhile? This condition makes me a failure at life. I'll never be able to achieve my goals and dreams because of how tired I am.*

- **Personalising** — Feeling responsible for things that are not your fault or incorrect assumptions around other people's responses being directed at you. It can lead to feelings such as indignation and choosing to take offence when none is meant.

  Examples: *I've done something wrong and it's my fault that I'm so tired. I'm not contributing as much as I used to with the household chores and my family resents me for it. My friends and family are angry at me as I don't support them as much as I used to. I hate how stressed everyone is at work and feel like it is directed at me.*

- **Filtering** — Bias in the way you see the world and looking for things that confirm your own prejudices, insecurities and fears.

  Examples: *My colleagues think I'm not pulling my weight because I only work my nominated hours and take my breaks. My friend is now angry at me as I didn't have the energy to attend their birthday party. I heard a family member say they're stressed and now I feel guilty for not being able to help them more with their workload.*

- **Blaming** — Assigning fault when dealing with unfavourable circumstances, mishaps, disappointments and mistakes. Blaming is usually oversimplistic and fails to acknowledge all the factors that contribute to outcomes. It creates feelings of anger, bitterness and resentment and prevents healing from taking place.

    Examples: *If only they had not attended that party, they would not have given me long-COVID. My doctor isn't doing enough to help me manage my fatigue. My manager is the reason why I'm so exhausted as they don't understand me. My partner just doesn't get it, which makes me feel even more exhausted.*

- **Comparing** — Comparing yourself to others, or even to a previous version of yourself, can lead to feeling inadequate.

    Examples: *Other people dealing with fatigue are handling it better than me. I used to be able to cope with my workload and now feel like I'm letting everyone down. I'm not as productive as my co-workers. I used to be on a path to success, but now I'm just on a path to failure.*

- **Just-world fallacy** — The assumption that things should be fair and that you live in an ideal world. It can lead to feeling angry and resentful.

    Examples: *It's not fair that I have this condition. I'm being punished for not living a healthy lifestyle. I must've done something wrong in the past to deserve feeling this exhausted. I'm angry that I'm no longer able to do the things I once could. It's not fair that it's so easy for others while everything is a struggle for me.*

What unhelpful thought patterns do you find yourself slipping into?

These thought patterns are certainly not kind and often not even rational as you fall victim to cognitive distortion. They can create a pessimistic or negative filter that distorts your reality. The result is often further exhaustion — exactly what you don't need when dealing with fatigue.

Our thought patterns are often so ingrained you won't even know you are employing distorted ways of thinking. As we have seen, they are usually a pattern from childhood, or even patterns you have picked up from others, such as friends, workmates or a life partner. You might find they are still being reinforced by the people in your inner circle.

Before moving to the next chapter, take some time to reflect on what your mindset around your condition truly looks like, including both the positive and negative thought patterns you hold. The next chapter will look at how to gain control of these thought patterns, managing the highs and the lows, and training your mind to promote healing and growth.

Putting it into practice

Take a moment to review your own mindset and thought patterns around your condition.

1. On good days, what thought patterns do you find helpful or supportive of your situation?
2. On darker days, what thought patterns do you find unhelpful or unsupportive of your situation?
3. What specific phrases can you identify that you use?
4. What have you heard others say that contributes to your own beliefs around your condition?
5. What are the differences you notice in your thinking on good and dark days?

Chapter 8
Developing a Healing Mindset

Pip was only 14 when she developed severe levels of fatigue after falling ill with a virus. Pip learnt the hard way that she had choices to make in managing both her energy and her mindset.

Not wanting to be left behind at school, she went through a period of trying to force herself to have more energy and attend her classes. Rather than resulting in more energy, it had the opposite effect. Pip became even more exhausted the next day than she would have been otherwise. She started feeling really down, like she was failing her parents, her friends and her teachers.

Pip soon realised that her mindset of 'forcing herself' was not working. She was only borrowing energy from her future, which she then had to pay back...with interest.

After seeing a local psychologist, Pip worked on her internal dialogue and her mood started lifting. This became a massive part of her eventual recovery. She ended up missing two terms of school, but rebounded to be able to start afresh the next year.

Looking back, Pip can see how it was pacing as well as easing the judgements she placed on herself that made all the difference. Only when the pressure was off did she start recovering. She stopped worrying about letting others down and forcing herself to carry on regardless, rather focusing on feeling healthy for the next day. This became a valuable lesson for her university days and the eventual launch of her (now very successful) career.

At the start of the unhelpful thinking discussion, we touched upon the topic of your mindset (your way of thinking around your fatigue condition), including both positive and negative elements.

You most likely saw how easy it can be to slip into unhelpful or negative thought patterns, especially when navigating a long-term condition like fatigue. Pip in the snapshot above demonstrates unhelpful thinking in action — **personalising** by thinking her condition was letting other people down and thinking she **should** be able to push through and attend her classes. This resulted in an unhealthy mindset that was not helping her fatigue — making it worse in fact. It was not until she saw a counsellor and worked on her mindset that she started to feel physical improvement.

This section looks at how you can transform those unhelpful thinking patterns into a more healing mindset.

A healing mindset is one of the best gifts you can give yourself as you travel through the highs and lows of long-term fatigue, or indeed any other long-term condition. You can't often control the reactions of others, but with practice you can control your thinking — the mindset and beliefs you hold around your condition.

A healing mindset refers to a way of thinking that promotes healing, growth and wellbeing. To overcome unhelpful programming, it focuses on helpful, constructive thoughts and actions. It provides nurture and support for your physical and emotional healing. It's about possibilities — hope for a positive future, rather than focusing only on your current situation.

My version of a healing mindset came out of my most difficult days. I worked with a psychologist who was able to assist me in expressing my frustrations and darkest feelings in a way that I never had before.

Speaking of psychology, this can be a touchy subject! Psychological interventions (such as cognitive behavioural therapy (CBT), acceptance and commitment therapy (ACT), emotion-focused therapy (EFT) or any other acronym you can throw at us) are not a treatment or cure for our underlying conditions. There are too many stories (including my own) where the physical side of the condition has been deemed too hard to handle or ignored. Instead, psychology becomes the magic panacea prescribed by ill-informed medical practitioners.

It's important to note that long-term fatigue conditions *are not* just psychosomatic, 'all in your head'. It isn't about sending you to a counsellor/psychologist/psychiatrist and all will be fine and dandy. These are complex conditions with many moving parts. They are not caused by being unfit or having a mental health condition.

Psychological interventions *can* however be helpful in supporting you to adjust and cope with your condition, putting you in the best possible mindset to heal.

My time with a psychologist was tremendously helpful, particularly around coping with what is an extremely challenging and long-term condition. It helped me better explain my condition to others. I was also more able to adjust to a new way of living and be okay with that —

eventually! — rather than drowning in despair. These are powerful tools for any of us to have in our toolbox.

And you know what? All this processing *did* have a good effect on my fatigue! I started noticing that my emotional state had a massive effect on how exhausted I was feeling. The mind-body connection meant that all my anxiety and despair, and all those times I labelled myself 'lazy', just fed my fatigue and resulted in exhaustion for days. I was draining my own energy. From this place, the strategies that made up my healing mindset started to form.

A healing mindset is not about adopting a Pollyanna personality, nor is it about positive thinking at all times. It's okay to feel complicated emotions like frustration, sadness, anger, fear or even despair. I certainly felt all of these and more. The secret is how long you sit in these negative emotions. You can acknowledge the difficult times, but the secret is not to dwell there indefinitely.

A healing mindset takes time and practice, catching yourself when you slip into internal name-calling or rumination for just that bit too long. I started small by implementing one rule — I needed to have a big belly laugh every day. I looked for the humour around me — in conversations, in the antics of my pups, in my choice of TV shows and movies. My healing mindset was based on lifting my own mood and allowing myself to find joy in my surroundings.

What would a healing mindset look like for you?

This section is about adding more tools to your toolbox, creating the best possible frame of mind to navigate long-term fatigue. You'll always have good days and bad, but a great question to ask is how you can encourage a positive mindset and manage the unhelpful thinking patterns identified in the previous chapter. Over time, you might even be able to access a more positive spin on the way you're living with long-term fatigue.

This section will look at five strategies that have really worked for me, traversing the marathon journey and arriving at my new normal.

- Strategy 1 — Mastering the art of the reframe
- Strategy 2 — Utilising productive conversations
- Strategy 3 — Letting go of what you cannot control
- Strategy 4 — Maintaining a strong sense of self
- Strategy 5 — Becoming your own hero

Finding your own variation of these strategies will ideally allow you to access a gentler path of self-compassion and resilience for yourself — your own healing mindset.

Strategy 1 — Mastering the art of the reframe

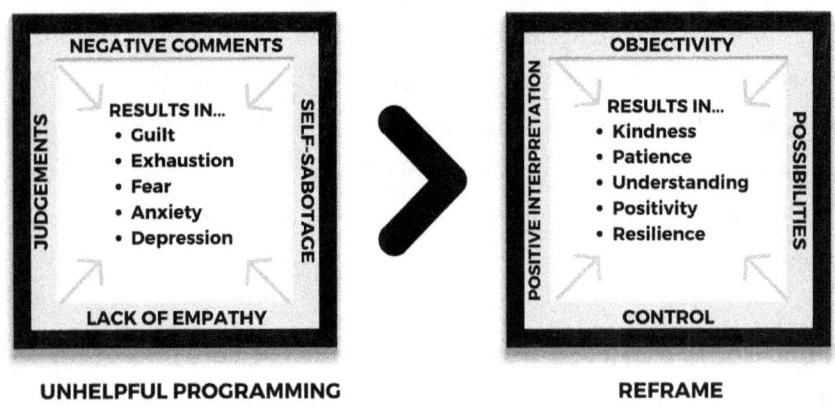

Figure 14 — Unhelpful Programming vs Reframing

Unhelpful programming starts with how you frame the way you look at the world — the perspective you take. When you look at different issues and events, you can make judgements and ascribe meaning based on your current frame of mind.

Reframing involves looking at that same issue or event in a new way or from another angle. A healing mindset is often about finding the angle that looks through a gentler, more generous or positive lens. It will feel less exhausting and abrasive and more uplifting.

Consider these two interpretations of the same facts:

- **Interpretation 1** — *'I went for a walk today and it was only 1000 steps. I used to be able to run 5km without breaking a sweat, so I'm feeling really disappointed in this effort. I've been in bed most of the week and expected so much more from myself.'*
- **Interpretation 2** — *'I went for a walk today and enjoyed it. It was 1000 steps. Considering I'd been in bed for most of this week, I see this as a win.'*

The facts are the same, but your interpretation or way of looking at them is completely different. Which way is easier? Which way is going to make you feel good about your situation? Which way is going to lead to recriminations and exhaustion?

Interpretation 1 is a good example of unhelpful programming in action. It is **comparing** what you used to be able to do with your current reality. It can be so tempting to compare. It is certainly natural to focus on the negative aspects of our struggle when affected by fatigue. However, Interpretation 2 is a good example of how you can reframe what presents itself to you, using a different way of thinking for a gentler, more compassionate view of the same situation.

What aspects of long-term fatigue can you reframe?

Reframing is a great tool for helping you better manage your emotions and the way you see even those darkest of days.

Different methods of reframing include:

a. **Objectivity**

   - Instead of emotion-driven thinking — *'Every minute of every day is awful.'*
   - Reframe by thinking less emotionally and more objectively — *'I recognise that for now some days will be difficult and some I'll have a bit more energy.'*

b. **Positive interpretation**

   - Instead of getting caught up in negativity and possibly catastrophising — *'I feel guilty, like I'm letting everyone down when I can't attend events.'*
   - Reframe by allowing a more positive interpretation — *'I'm not able to make these events right now, but those close to me will empathise and understand as I communicate my challenges.'*

c. **Focus on possibilities**

   - Instead of focusing on what is *not* possible right now — *'My team expects me to work full-time. I am not able to right now and I feel like I'm letting them down.'*
   - Reframe to focus on what *is* possible — *'I am able to work part-time, and this allows me to bring my best self to support my team, without stressing me out mentally and physically.'*

d. **Impact what's within your control**
   - Instead of feeling like things are outside your control — *'I feel helpless, like nothing I do has any impact. This is going to ruin my life.'*
   - Reframe to specific action that you can do something about — *'I'm going to do what my body dictates for now, also giving myself time to rest and recover.'*

I've found the result of reframing to be a mindset that is kinder and more positive in perspective. Reframing can also foster more patience with your situation. You're bound to still have those bad days, but reframing may help you feel more able to cope and/or less stressed when they do happen. I've also found it the key to building greater resilience around how to manage your condition over the long-term.

Strategy 2 — Utilising productive conversations

When experiencing more negative emotions around long-term fatigue, the next strategy involves using what I call 'productive conversations'.

Productive conversations are when you become more analytical and work through your experience rather than just venting. This can be either:

- **Internally**, through your own thoughts or other methods such as journaling. Sometimes even sleeping on it can result in waking with a clearer frame of mind.
- **With someone else**, such as a trusted friend or family member. It can also be a trained professional such as a counsellor or psychologist.

Now, don't get me wrong, I'm all for venting! One of the worst things you can do is to gloss over your negative emotions. When you're living with long-term fatigue, negative emotions such as frustration, sadness, loneliness and anger are bound to come up. These are real feelings. The grief cycle shows us this forms part of a natural process.

It's healthy to acknowledge rather than suppress these emotions. If you do tend to suppress them, you run the risk of the same emotions bubbling up again and again without them actually being resolved. Acknowledging honestly and openly what you are feeling can help you process and work through the full range of emotions you are experiencing.

It can also feel good to vent and have someone listen. It serves to bring you closer to that person, building stronger bonds and helping you feel less alone because you know there are people in this world seeking to understand. It is, however, helpful to recognise there is a fine line between venting and complaining, too much of which can push people away.

Like so many, I was 'expressing' (okay venting!) a bit too much at the beginning of my exhausting journey. It can feel impossible to be calm and considered when you are not sure what is happening to your body, mind or even your sanity! At first, I felt furious when others didn't want to engage. Couldn't they see how much I was hurting? My raw, unprocessed emotions were just too much for certain people to handle. Eventually, I had to accept that venting was just serving to make them uncomfortable and me frustrated.

Over time, I did find sympathetic audiences, including people in like-minded Facebook groups and supportive professionals, both of which helped process my more difficult emotions in a safe setting.

Pure venting also doesn't do anything to reframe the experience. In fact, it can do the opposite — further embedding those negative beliefs and often resulting in feeling even worse than when you started. What you don't want to do is to experience negative emotions indefinitely.

This is where those productive conversations can become a key part of your healing mindset. You will gradually find that balance of how to communicate your experience to others for greater understanding. You will also be able to experience the more difficult negative emotions, but not sit and wallow in them indefinitely. Rather, you can process your emotions and eventually employ the first strategy — reframing.

> >> There is an art to expressing yourself in a way that the other person is able to receive. If you're struggling to communicate your experience with those around you, I have channelled my experiences into a free e-book that provides advice and scripts around how to spark these types of productive conversations.
>
> You can find this here — www.sarahvizer.com/tootiredtothink

What does a productive conversation involve?

Different outcomes of a productive conversation include the following:

a. **You process your emotions rather than just sitting or wallowing in them** — e.g. Rather than just feeling frustrated, you identify that the frustration arises from feeling like you are not able to do a certain activity. Instead, you reframe this into what you *can do* right now.

b. **You can openly share your experiences and feel validated** — e.g. Rather than just venting about how tired you're feeling and how no one can understand, you talk through your feelings resulting in a sense of validation and connection with the other person because they really do come to understand the impact of your tiredness.

c. **You can analyse deeper feelings** — e.g. You go deeper and seek to understand more analytically the root of your feelings, such as anger arising from a fear of not ever seeing improvement in your condition.

d. **You identify how you dealt with similar issues in the past** — e.g. When stressed in the past, you've had similar issues with brain fog and helped resolve it by writing lists, utilising your diary and cutting back your expectations for yourself.

e. **You can break out of negativity and enter a more solution-oriented frame of mind** — e.g. Rather than ruminating over a missed opportunity, such as not being able to attend an important event, you are able to develop a new approach for the next time the opportunity arises. This may be blocking out the days before and strictly resting ahead of the event.

f. **You can stay focused on the topic at hand and avoid getting sidetracked** — e.g. When talking to a friend, you stay focused on your main issues around fatigue rather than getting sidetracked with other worries or concerns (which can quickly lead to overwhelm).

When was the last time you felt like you had a productive conversation?

You know the conversation has been productive when you feel better, more in control and like you are on a healing path. You still receive all the benefits of stronger bonds and feeling less alone, but you also know you are building your resources and energy through your conversations rather than embedding the negativity.

It really doesn't matter if it's with someone else or just a conversation you have with yourself. Each of these outcomes allows you to acknowledge and not suppress the inevitable negative emotions that show up. You are then better able to process the emotion and circle back to that first strategy — the reframe.

Strategy 3 — Letting go of what you cannot control

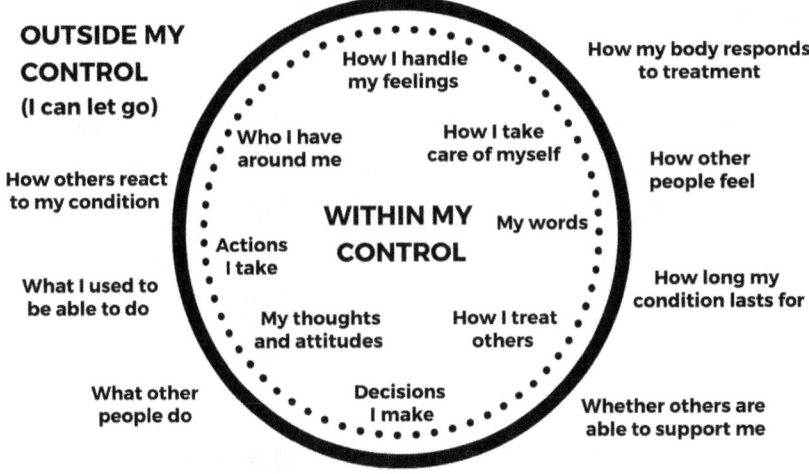

Figure 15 — Within My Control vs Outside My Control

We've now recognised that dealing with long-term fatigue can be the most frustrating and challenging experience to go through. And that's putting it mildly!

One of these sources of frustration is that there are numerous factors over which you have absolutely no control. It's quite easy to get stuck in a pattern of thinking that results in you ruminating over issues such as:

- How long you'll be affected
- The unfairness of other people not understanding your condition
- How much you used to be able to do versus what you can do now
- Feeling stuck with fatigue that just won't go away no matter what you do

- How to get others to support you in the ways that you want them to

The list goes on!

Emotions like frustration are a waste of your precious energy! You might notice how all the points above correspond to factors outside of the circle in Figure 16. These are factors that you cannot change; they are outside your influence and control.

A better use of your energy is to focus on what's firmly within your control. A bit like the serenity prayer, you want to acknowledge the things you cannot change (those outside the circle). You might prefer they go a different way, but have no actual say over the outcome. Instead, you'll focus your energy on the things you can change and do have control over (those inside the circle).

You'll probably still have moments of frustration, stress, disappointment and so on, but the goal of a healing mindset is to focus on how best to use your valuable energy.

Let's look at some examples of how you can use your mindset training to bring things back into your control.

OUT OF YOUR CONTROL (FRUSTRATION, STRESS, DISAPPOINTMENT MINDSET)	WITHIN YOUR CONTROL (HEALING MINDSET)
INSTEAD OF: I rested all day and still don't have the energy to cook a meal tonight - it's so frustrating.	**OPTION:** I saved my energy and enjoyed an evening of rest by ordering a food delivery. I'm at peace with this.
INSTEAD OF: I've tried all the recommended medical treatments, but my fatigue remains stubbornly present - it's so disappointing.	**OPTION:** I accept that I've done everything possible for now to help my condition. I'm focussing on letting it go.
INSTEAD OF: I've explained my limited energy as best as I can to a close friend and they still do not understand. They keep inviting me to events I cannot attend - it's so stressful.	**OPTION:** I now smile when my friend invites me. I thank them for thinking of me and remind them that I have limited energy and most likely will not be able to attend, but I'm grateful they include me.

Table 4 — Within Your Control and a Healing Mindset

You might notice common themes in the examples above and how you go about developing a healing mindset — being at peace with your decisions, letting go and feeling positive emotions such as gratitude. These are all the hallmarks of **acceptance** — the end point of your grief cycle rollercoaster of emotions.

Bringing things into your control and your healing mindset is about:

a. **Feeling at peace** with the actions you have taken and letting go of the outcome
b. **Letting go** of what drains your energy and causes frustration, stress or disappointment
c. **Accepting** that things won't always go your way
d. **Communicating your boundaries** to others then leaving it at that, no matter the outcome
e. **Allowing other people to react** in the way they choose but keeping your own peace of mind intact

Strategy 4 — Maintaining a strong sense of self

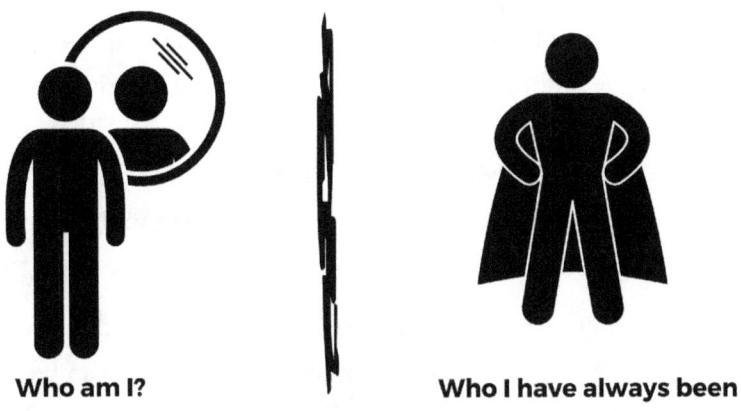

Figure 16 — Maintaining a Strong Sense of Self

When you are dealing with a long-term condition like fatigue, it can be that you start to align your identity to that illness or condition. It can become all-consuming, especially if you start to define yourself solely in terms of the condition. You might even find yourself identifying as a 'sick person' rather than who you actually are at your core.

Here are two examples that demonstrate this:

- **Fatigue becomes the dominant aspect of your personality** — You define yourself as a ME/CFS, fibromyalgia or long-COVID sufferer over anything else that defines you. You might say things like, *"I used to be… Now I have long-COVID."*
- **You define yourself by your limitations** — You tell people what you cannot do rather than what you can do. When someone asks you to do any activity, your go-to response becomes, *"No, I can't do that… I have ME/CFS."*

Not only do you define yourself by these newer limitations, but you might even start to think less of yourself because of your condition. This is where those unhelpful thought patterns can kick right back in, impeding your progress as you navigate your marathon journey.

Your condition will most likely have brought about changes — physical, lifestyle, cognitive and social changes. Your goals and priorities may have moved and you're likely to be feeling limitations right now. These changes will mean there will be activities you can no longer do, relationships that are altered, even structural changes in life - such as needing to live somewhere new or changes to your work situation.

Feelings of grief and loss around these changes can kick off the grief process, even grieving for the person you used to be. Your grief can be cyclical too; when you find yourself traversing Kübler-Ross' grief cycle in this way, you may feel acceptance for the changes one day, then thrown back into anger or depression the next.

Considering this is a long-term, often hidden condition that stops you from being able to fully share the experience with others in a way they understand, this grief you feel is real and valid. However, none of this changes who you are at your core.

I've come to realise that these conditions are *happening to you*, not something you *are*. You are still the same person you have always been. That is what you can trust — that is **the true you**. You are not the circumstances around what you are currently experiencing. You have the same strengths, the same accomplishments. You are still that same person.

Chronic fatigue syndrome had a massive impact on my sense of self and identity. I am an energetic, vital person, so at times I didn't recognise the person staring back at me in the mirror. I felt robbed of the energy and vitality that I was so used to seeing. I was constantly surprised that my partner Demian saw my inner energy, particularly when I felt so tired!

What he was seeing was my essence shining through. It took me a while to trust in this, but when I did, I felt like myself again, even when I was affected by fatigue. While my outlook on life may have changed, I was the same person I'd always been.

Over time, I learnt to acknowledge the grief, the frustration at my current limitations, the anger at the changes I was forced to make totally outside my control. It was still frustrating on occasion, but overall I shifted my mindset to stop defining myself by these changes. I no longer placed my chronic fatigue condition at the centre of my day. I realised I was indulging in unhelpful thought processes like comparison and just-world fallacy with the result of making myself miserable.

Instead, I found trust that I was the same person I'd always been. My go-to emotion became acceptance towards what I *could* do on any given day. When I start to feel frustration (which does still happen mind you) I acknowledge the loss but remind myself that I'm not going to define myself by my condition or daily achievements. Maintaining a strong sense of self has helped me through the harder times and formed part of my healing mindset.

This strategy is about building trust in your identity, even enlisting support when you need it from those who know you well to remind you, '*I see you*'. It might feel hard to trust right now but know that your true essence is shining through. It may simply not be visible to you right now. The traits that define you are all still there; they just may not be so apparent as you focus on rest, recharge and recovery.

Strategy 5: Becoming your own hero

The last strategy, becoming your own hero, is about empowering you to take ownership of your situation.

It can be tempting to fall into powerlessness, feeling like you are not in control, screwed over by relentless fatigue and the various struggling medical systems.

I get it!

While I'm sure we all have moments of this, how disempowering does it feel to view your situation through this lens? It's setting you up to feel more stress and anxiety, maybe even hurting your self-esteem. It also adds to the levels of fatigue you're already feeling.

You do not need to stay strong every minute of every day. People like us all have periods of time when long-term fatigue can feel overwhelming or another of the negative emotions that are part of that grief cycle. You might even descend into an inevitable pity party. *'Why is this happening to me?'* was a common thought I had navigating fatigue day-in, day-out. These are the days when you do not feel like a hero at all.

What would be a better way? My healing mindset is not about never having these days. Rather it becomes about how you can get yourself through them. With a healing mindset, you can work towards getting faster at pulling yourself out. I'm very good at allowing myself a little time in the pity zone, but I'm getting increasingly better at deciding it's now time to move forwards. Often my overnight sleep is what's needed for this reset to occur.

This sense of forward momentum is my own superpower. Becoming your own hero is about helping your healing mindset by tapping into that unstoppable will to move forward — finding your own superpowers.

How do you become your own hero and tap into these powers? A few ways include:

1. **Keeping perspective**
    - Empowering yourself to keep on going and stay focused on your own healing
    - Taking each day as it comes and maintaining perspective on your bad days — finding hope that the future will be brighter
    - Getting quicker at pulling yourself out of the low times

2. **Advocating for yourself**
    - Educating yourself on how best to help your long-term fatigue
    - Using your voice and not letting anyone else speak for you

3. **Building support**
   - Finding the team that can give you the support you need right now
   - Utilising members of your team to help validate your view of who you are and the acknowledgement that, '*I see you*', can bring

4. **Taking action**
   - Taking action as best you can to manage your situation
   - When something isn't working, finding something else that will

As the hero of your story, your healing mindset comes from feeling that you are in charge of the decisions you make. This can be any decision, such as what treatment you take, who you have around you or what life looks like for you.

You and you alone can take ownership and be the hero of your own story!

Eventually, you might even find something meaningful emerges from your experience, as described in the sixth phase of the grief cycle.

Pulling it together

These five strategies have supported me immensely over my marathon journey, helping create what's become my new normal. They can be used individually or in combination to develop a mindset that is less around angst and more around self-compassion, resilience and forward momentum — your own version of a healing mindset.

In the opening snapshot, Pip certainly demonstrated Strategy 3 in action — letting go of what she could not control. Being only 14 at the time, she was also able to internalise some helpful lessons early in life, creating a strong sense of self that did not include her fatigue as a defining characteristic (Strategy 4).

My own experience with Strategy 5, becoming my own hero, has been particularly life-changing. While I still have my moments, my feelings of powerlessness were mostly transformed to empowerment when I started writing this book and recording our shared experiences. There's something to be said for knowing you're not alone in this experience that feels truly transformative.

In some ways, this is the most crucial part of the whole equation — finding the strategies that work for you. The end goal becomes about learning how to proactively manage your frame of mind, rather than reactively responding to each situation. This section is relevant not just for managing long-term fatigue, but any challenge you face in life.

Using these tools over time, you can expect to experience a more optimistic and proactive approach to your healing journey, even if you still have those bad spells. The next section offers some good advice around how others navigate these low periods, ones I've come to know as my dark days.

Putting it into practice

Spend a moment reviewing the five strategies and how you can use each one to develop a more healing mindset.

1. How can you **reframe something happening in your life right now** to take a more compassionate view? Try reframing it in a few different ways:

    a. Objectivity
    b. Positive interpretation
    c. Focus on possibilities
    d. Impact what's within your control

2. Thinking of something that is bothering you, what outcomes do you need from a productive conversation? With this in mind, how can your next conversation become more **productive**?

Tip: It can be with someone else or internally with yourself.

   a. Do you want to **process emotions** and reframe them for next time?
   b. Will you **share your experiences** to create mutual understanding?
   c. Can you delve below the surface of a negative emotion, and **analyse** the cause and its impact on you?
   d. Do you wish to draw on past experiences to **find patterns**, then form strategies to deal with current issues?
   e. Do you need to **solve a problem**?
   f. Are you trying to **focus deeply** on an important topic, rather than listing all your worries and adding to overwhelm?

3. What would you like to let go of that's **out of your control** and focus more on that's **within your control**?

4. Where does your true self shine through? Outline how you can maintain a strong **positive sense of self** and not align yourself too closely to your condition.

5. How can you take more ownership of your situation and **become your own hero**? List how you can:

   a. Keep perspective
   b. Advocate for yourself
   c. Build support
   d. Take action

Chapter 9
Preparing for Those Dark Days

Ben, a 32-year-old engineer living in Singapore, is now in his 18th month of a ME/CFS diagnosis. He has a strained relationship with work, which has been experiencing an unprecedented busy time. He also feels strained with his parents, who pressure him to engage more with his family.

Ben's body, mind and heart are at complete odds. He desperately wants to honour his commitments and finds himself pushing harder than what's advisable at work to make sure he delivers. This comes at great cost. Last month, he pushed too hard, resulting in a crash that eclipsed all crashes before. He was literally not able to get out of bed for days.

Ben felt a complex mix of shame, despair and heartache when this happened. He was stuck at home, feeling lonely and isolated and lacking the support he needs at work and from his family.

Something has to give. Ben doesn't want to go through such an emotionally intensive period again without having a plan in place to manage these complex emotions. He is preparing to have some difficult yet productive conversations with both work and his family to take some of the pressure off. He is also looking for ways to feel more connected with others when he is going through a crash and stuck at home in bed.

So far, we've looked at how to identify unhelpful programming when it slips in and train your mind to make a different choice — a gentler, more healing way of thinking. This may sound straightforward, but it can be extremely difficult to action.

You've seen there will be peaks and troughs during your time of healing. Some days your energy kicks in and you feel on top of the world; on those days, it's a lot easier to employ this healing mindset. But it's the others - the days when you have little to no energy that can plunge you into the depths of despair. They can kick you straight back into those unhelpful thinking patterns. Let's call these your **dark days**.

This is our emotional reality. Dark days will occur. The question is: how can you be as prepared as possible to make them slightly less dark, moving yourself into the light?

I've had many dark days, and if I'm honest, I still do on occasion. There are some days where it just feels impossible to control my mindset and I sink into foggy feelings of despair. I've come to recognise these feelings as temporary, and over the years become much faster at pulling myself out of these less-than-helpful emotions.

You might implement all the strategies outlined in the last chapter and still find these days difficult to navigate. So, what else can you do when you have a dark day?

The focus for this section is based on the reality that there will be some dark days ahead when dealing with long-term fatigue. You can come prepared with a goal and strategies to place to help yourself deal with these tougher times.

What are your goals for navigating the dark days?

Your goals are simple statements that summarise what you want to achieve.

Ben in the opening snapshot had several goals, a summary of which could be:

1. Find ways to remove the pressure that leads to physical crashes
2. Learn how to better handle complex emotions, such as shame, despair and heartache
3. Enlist more support at work and from family
4. Mitigate feeling lonely and isolated when lacking energy and stuck at home through greater emotional connection

You can see from Ben's examples that goals are around the pain points or problem areas you're feeling. If you can identify those areas to improve, you'll know what strategies to have in place to make these days just a little less dark.

To create your own set of goals, have a think about these three questions:

1. **What are the pain points you want to address?** e.g. times of pressure and/or overwhelm, specific unhelpful thinking patterns, building greater awareness of triggers, feeling unsupported, experiencing a lack of connection, developing a more positive mindset around how the condition is being handled.

2. **What is the outcome you want to achieve?** e.g. feeling calmer and more relaxed, cultivating a daily self-care routine, building a toolbox of healthy coping strategies.
3. **Who else do you need to involve?** e.g. growing a stronger support network, developing greater understanding from people around you, enlisting professional support such as a psychologist.

From these questions, examples of specific goals you may have for your dark days include:

- Identifying specific activities I will and won't do on my dark days
- Having a predefined list of methods for lowering expectations of myself when I start to experience signs such as pressure or overwhelm
- Understanding what triggers my unhelpful thinking patterns and developing ways to mitigate this
- Having a toolkit of three strategies in place for when I feel…(insert your own emotion here)
- Identifying methods to keep my relationships intact and not take out my frustration on others
- Enlisting more understanding and support from…(insert your list of people and professional support here)
- Getting better at strategies around living in the present moment, rather than focusing on the future or the past
- Learning how to surrender to my dark days and not waste my energy trying to 'fight' the feeling

There's a lot to work with here, so my best advice would be to start with a simple goal and build from there. In the early days of my fatigue, my goal focused mainly on finding strategies to keep me afloat when struck with those all-too-familiar feelings of overwhelm and frustration. Ideally, you can start small, concentrating on your own pain points and what will provide maximum benefit in your situation.

Based on your goal, what strategies will you put in place?

Once you have established your pain points and goals for your dark days, you can look for some strategies to put in place for these days to shine just that little bit brighter.

How can you do this? Here are some suggestions around how others have navigated their own dark days of fatigue.

*"On those really dark days, I let myself **have a good cry**. I used to cry once every six months, but since having long-COVID, I cry on average about once a week. It's okay — it's my release and I've learnt to allow it and say to myself each time that crying is nature's tranquiliser. After a good crying session, I feel like an empty vessel that I can then start to fill up again, stacking new emotions that make me feel stronger and more in control."*

*"I tend to feel overwhelmed sometimes. I've always had a tendency towards anxious thinking, ruminating on one thing after another until I feel really worked up. When my body aches and I have all these other things wrong, it just amplifies my anxiety to the point of absolute exhaustion. When things become overwhelming, I now **write a list of what's on my mind** and then consciously **relax my body and tell myself I'm going to sleep on it**. Trying to deal with all these spiralling emotions in one day is too much to manage, but waking up to a new day somehow clears my slate. I can look at that list and sometimes even wonder what I was so worried about!"*

"It's taken me a while (think eight months!) but I've now **set up a great support network to help when I feel down**. I even have a name for it: 'Phone a lifeline!' I have three friends who I've had long conversations with and understand. They are all happy to take a call on those days when I'm going through it. I used to feel like I was burdening them, but after asking directly I can see they are happy to have something they can do to help. I also have a psychologist who I speak to once a month via Zoom. I still have those days, but since having my lifelines in place, dealing with those doomsday emotions has become exponentially easier."

"Breathing is what gets me through. Dealing with chronic fatigue syndrome is so hard mentally, but a gamechanger was **learning 'box breathing'**. You start by counting…breathing in for 4, holding for 4, then breathing out for 4. I lie on my bed and put my hand on my stomach, pushing the air so deep down that my stomach pushes on my hand as it rises then falls again. I do this for a few minutes and find it so relaxing. It helps send oxygen around my body and calms everything down. I often find myself slipping into sleep from here. It's a lifesaver when my body is aching from tiredness."

"I've learnt how to **mindfully point my focus towards signs of improvement** rather than dwelling on what feels bad. I used to feel hopeless, like things would never improve. Like a child growing, when you live with fatigue daily, you don't always notice the little signs of recovery that are present along the way. These are things like not getting as much PEM after an event, feeling energised not drained after a great conversation, being able to read for 20 minutes etc. I've learnt to ride the positive wave and acknowledge any signs of improvement I see. On my darkest days, I then have something to hold onto."

"There are days I feel vulnerable and hypersensitive. On those days, I often need to **get back in bed and just ride it out**. There will then come a point in the day that I feel less vulnerable, stronger and more in control. It's that feeling that I wait for. It makes me feel like I've achieved something that day. I've faced down the worst of my demons and made it through. I have hope that the next day I will be a little stronger and things will be a little better."

"Some days are just awful, and I know on these days I need to **focus solely on self-care**. My husband takes the kids to school, and I set zero expectations for myself. I used to constantly run around, trying to keep everyone else happy in this family, but they have adapted quite well and are now far more self-sufficient. I still have my moments of guilt, but in so many ways long-COVID has helped me **rediscover who I am** and taught me a valuable lesson around how to properly look after myself."

"There are days when visual mediums like reading or TV are just too exhausting and I can only **listen to music or an entertaining podcast**. I have a playlist ready to go for these occasions — a soothing selection of music which also has upbeat lyrics. I also have my go-to podcasts — either comedy or inspirational interviews."

"I watch my language on my dark days and **put distance between what I'm feeling and who I identify as.** An example is when I'm feeling tired and frustrated. Check out the difference between these two sentences:

- Blaming myself: 'I'm so tired and frustrated.'
- Keeping distance: 'This tiredness is frustrating.'

It's subtle, but rather than saying 'I'm' and relating it directly to myself, I keep distance from the negative feelings. I find it helps me keep *objectivity around my situation, rather than sinking into the negative emotion."*

*"Over the years I've **developed my own language** around what I'm feeling, particularly when it's really bad. Now all I need to say is that I'm 'critical' and the whole household jumps to action clearing the path so I can lie down. They know I don't use this often, but when I do it means I'm at the end of my resilience for that day and need to immediately rest in a dark room. I've heard of others having their own words for this feeling that they can use at both home and in their workplace. It helps."*

These are just a few of the strategies available to you and there are so many more that you could use to help manage your darkest of days. A good practice is to have a strategy bank built up ahead of time that you can refer to when you are critically short on energy and need a quick solution.

With all this in place, there is one final and extremely important topic to consider in your emotional reality — managing the people in your life.

Putting it into practice

Spend a moment considering those dark days, the problem areas you can identify (from which you will develop your goals) and the methods you'll use to make them that little bit more manageable (strategies).

1. **What are your goals for dark days?**

    a. What are the pain points you want to address?
    b. What is the outcome you want to achieve?
    c. Who else do you need to involve?

2. **What are your strategies for dark days?** Spend a bit of time now creating your strategy bank to help you address your goals.

Tip: *The help section will also support you in developing strategies. You may want to come back and add to your strategy bank once you've read that section.*

Chapter 10

Managing the People in Your Life

David is a 58-year-old associate law professor who worked for a prestigious US university. He's currently on leave after battling the effects of long-COVID for three years and recently has found his relationship with his wife reaching a crisis point.

David has a number of fatigue symptoms, including POTS and PEM. He battles dizziness and nausea when travelling in a car for more than a few minutes. He's seen several doctors over the years but got to the point where he gave up after they failed to provide assistance that worked. He felt he was wasting his time, money and energy.

From his wife's point of view, David is not trying hard enough, his symptoms are an excuse and he should be having more tests done, or at least keep trying to help himself. Even though David is home all day, his wife works and does most of the household chores as well as taking their children to their events.

It's a difficult situation for both David and his wife. David has channelled his writing talents to put some of his frustrations down on paper, explaining to his wife more clearly how he is feeling and what is happening to his body. She has been open to reading and listening to his point of view. He has committed to looking for a more proactive solution, even consulting with a long-COVID clinic that has recently opened in their town.

Despite making progress, both remain cautious and unsure where their marriage is heading. David is working up to having necessary conversations with his wife, which can be extra difficult when he is feeling so fatigued, but are important. He is committed to having productive conversations that will bring him greater support and his wife less angst around the situation.

Who you have around you is so important to your health and happiness at the best of times, but even more important when you are experiencing long-term fatigue.

It's challenging to explain to others what it's like living life when you don't have energy and vitality. This is especially true if you once were a highly energetic person.

Recently, I had a conversation with a friend who asked me what our most valuable resource was. *"Easy, energy,"* I replied instantly. I was puzzled when he shook his head. *"Okay, energy and health,"* I suggested. Again, no. Seriously, what could be more important than our health and our energy? *"Time,"* he responded.

We all have different perspectives, and I could see that was true for his set of circumstances, but for anyone dealing with long-term fatigue, *energy* is likely to be the ultimate resource and *time* can actually become an enemy.

Getting through the day often feels like a mammoth effort. If anything, on some days, I could do with less time to have to get through!

It struck me then that I'd been trying to explain my condition to this friend for years, but still he had not quite got it. His perception of me was stuck in the past, at the vital energetic person I once was. The words 'chronic fatigue syndrome' might not mean much to him, but to me they were everything.

Looking for a diagnosis is one of the first things you will likely do. With this in place, it becomes so much more than mere words. It's an explanation, a way of getting help and a conduit to connecting with others.

Having a diagnosis and some understanding around your condition gives you more information to pass on to those around you. Yet it still doesn't guarantee that they will *understand* your condition. Continually explaining yourself and your circumstances can be a thankless and exhausting process!

Keeping your relationships energy positive

As humans, we are wired to seek connection and understanding. You saw in the pacing section that the way you 'spend' your energy each day is important. Understanding your limits and conserving your energy for what you most need to do in the day can become the priority.

Keeping your current relationships as **energy positive** as possible is the best-case scenario. This is my golden rule of energy – only doing what brings you more energy than you are required to spend – and this also extends to people. Of course, this requires you to be aware of the energy you expend in relationships.

GOLDEN RULE OF ENERGY

To only do things or have interactions which give you more energy than they require from you.

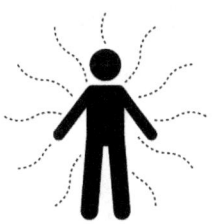

Figure 17 — My Golden Rule of Energy

Now, you can't control every interaction and person you will meet. You might find medical appointments frustrating but necessary. Your workmates or family probably won't always meet the golden rule. In general, though, where you have control over who's in your environment, the golden rule helps keep you focused on those energy positive relationships.

For a long time, my dog was the only 'person' I could be around for any length of time. He listened, let me cry and never passed judgement! Gradually, my energy started allowing more engagement with human company.

When you're depleted, previously reciprocal relationships — at work, or a friendship or close family members — may need to become more about you as you make sense of what's happening to you. The issue with long-term fatigue is people can be understanding of one-way relationships for only so long. This can create tension in even the tightest of relationships.

Having been a giving person and with a lifetime of doing all the right things under my belt, it was difficult for me to focus solely on myself for a while. It felt like I was being selfish and that felt wrong. Really, it was the only way I was able to heal. Like the team tells you in the safety briefing of any aircraft, you need to put on your own oxygen mask before you can assist others. You can only hope that your key relationships will last the distance.

What types of relationships do you have around you?

I've found that relationships you've developed over time can go in one of a few directions. I've categorised these into three groups!

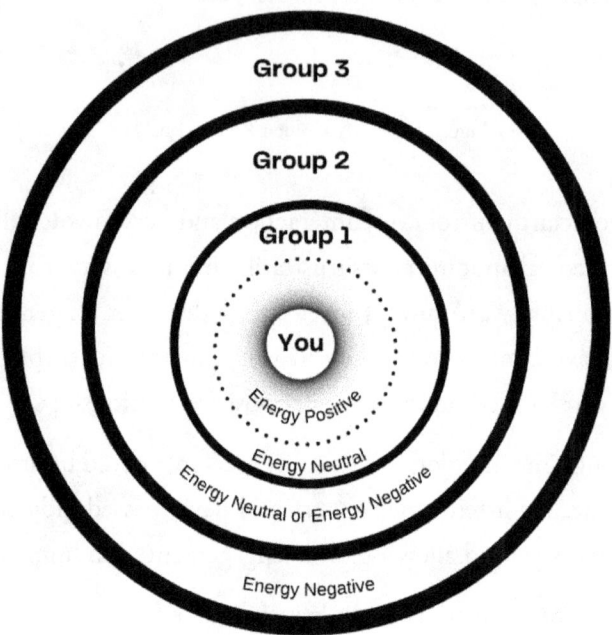

Figure 18 - Relationship Groups

- **Group 1 — People want to understand and help.** These are your energy neutral people, as they have good intentions, but might not fully grasp your condition or provide the support you actually need. The ones who are actively able to help in the right ways are your energy positive people.

- **Group 2 — People leave you alone as you become too much to handle.** These relationships can suffer. It will depend on how much you have to give as to whether they last the distance.

- **Group 3 — People actively set you back.** These are your doubters, medical professionals who gaslight or people who just cannot understand your condition. These become your energy negative people. Where possible, you may choose to disengage.

Let's look at each group in turn.

Group 1
People who want to understand and help
Even though you have less energy to give, you most likely will need support more than ever during this time. Some relationships will step up and be the heroes that you need right now. These people will make efforts to understand your situation, or at least give you the space that you need.

These relationships are the ones most likely to be worth the expenditure of your precious energy.

Be aware that you are also part of other people's orbit. What role do you play? Are you giving them the time, attention, energy, concern, wisdom they require? The best relationships have their periods of give and take.

You might not have the resources to play the role you have previously. You might be less available, more emotional, less able to physically meet, less able to have intense or negative conversations.

You can outline your challenges by engaging in productive conversations, which also form part of your healing mindset. Productive conversations with others where you outline your situation as clearly as you can will hopefully help both of you understand each other's needs and position.

Sometimes new relationships are required. Strangers in online groups or people loosely in your social circle may take less energy expenditure than close friends while still providing a sense of community.

Finally, consider the paid professional who can help and find your team of supportive practitioners. In the medical reality section, we will see that a good place to start is to build your relationship with your primary care doctor who can then help you build your team of practitioners.

Who do you have in your Group 1?

Action to take:

- Invest in these relationships
- Actively have productive conversations
- Know that new relationships may be required — e.g. online support groups
- Find your team of supportive professional practitioners

Group 2
People who leave you alone or disappear completely

Dealing with your condition, your lack of energy and other symptoms, and the highs and lows they bring may be too much for some people. Some of your current relationships will suffer and potentially not survive.

One aspect to be aware of is that your condition might change the rules or your way of interacting with others. In my case, I went from being extroverted and energetic to being touchy, introverted and frequently wanting to be left alone. It was nothing anyone had said or done; my energy was depleted, and I had literally nothing left to give.

Your feelings can also become amplified as you deal with the negative aspects of your condition. Quite simply, the focus of the relationship might need to be mainly about you for a while.

All of this brings changes that can have a jarring effect on those around you — close and more distant.

Examples of these changes include:

- A previously positive, happy person may morph into a sad, depressed hermit, who struggles to come out of their room
- A normally positive, can-do attitude at work starts to become negative, even angry, as the person looks for ways to do less work
- A usually patient, kind individual starts to snap regularly, even getting a good dose of rage

What other changes have you noticed?
These examples of change are quite understandable when dealing with long-term fatigue, but you can probably start see how these changes could upset others and even result in them avoiding such company.

It can depend on how receptive and understanding others are to your condition as to whether your current relationships last the distance. Of course, it also depends on the other person's bandwidth. The challenges they are facing can mean they don't have the energy themselves to support you in the ways that you need right now.

When this happens and people disappear from your life, it can be disappointing and hurt…a lot. I know.

Spending energy mourning these relationships, wishing it was a different way, even trying to change the outcome can be energetically expensive. I found that railing against the lack of support only served to torment both of us.

Learning to let go of relationships, even for just a while, can be one of the hardest things to face. Paradoxically, once you do let go, it can be exactly what frees you to spend your energy on yourself and develop the relationships you really do need right now. It can save you countless sleepless nights and energy drain.

When it's limited, your energy is an investment. Learning when your investment in relationships is worth it or when you need to call it quits is a lifelong challenge.

Who do you have in your Group 2?

Action to take:

- Conserve your energy within these relationships
- Employ productive conversations to try to convert Group 2 into Group 1
- Learn to let go, even if it's just for a while
- View your energy as an investment and invest wisely!

Group 3
People who actively set you back

Energy is needed to maintain relationships. Often, you can't do that well when you have so little energy to give. It's important to be aware of energy drain and the different people who influence your energy.

Sooner or later, we realise that positive and negative emotions are catching. A smile and kind word are catching; so too are stress and overwhelm. There's even a term for it — **emotional contagion**[28]. If you're surrounded by stressed-out people, chances are you will also be stressed-out. Listening to

---

[28] A good example of both positive and negative emotional contagion is outlined in the 2021 article by Jeffrey Gaines, Ph.D. titled, 'What is emotional contagion theory? (definition and examples). Article link - positivepsychology.com/emotional-contagion/

other people's problems can become an absolute drain on your energy bank. Even the most resilient of us can be worn down by that over time.

Another topic to be aware of is all the unsolicited advice floating around and how draining it can be on you as the receiver. Whenever you bring up fatigue, it might seem like everyone has the secret answer, the magic bullet. If I'd implemented all the unsolicited solutions and advice received over the years, I'd be both broke and exhausted!

Group 3 people are energetically expensive. These are the ones that require the most energy and leave you with less energy than when you started — they break the golden rule! As much as possible, you'll want to move these relationships from energy negative to either being energy neutral, or in the best case, energy positive.

Sometimes, however, this is just not possible. It could be you don't bring out the best in each other or there's sources of tension, spoken or otherwise. In this scenario, it can be that your best option is limiting your time or disengaging completely with the relationships that actively set you back. This might be for a while or even forever. As the saying goes: *"People come into your life for a reason, a season or a lifetime."*

This becomes difficult when you are tethered to them in some way, such as close family, neighbours, people in your workplace etc. When this is the case, what you can do is be aware of the effect they have on your energy and make choices.

Choices can be around spending less time than you normally would with these people. You can work on techniques that protect you, such as boundary-setting and setting up a forcefield to 'protect' your energy.

In the medical reality section, you will see the strong need to advocate for yourself with your practitioners. Medical doctors like to heal and can become frustrated with any lack of progress. They can even gaslight you into thinking it's all in your head, or something you should be dealing with better. They are wrong and practitioners who are not helpful need to be replaced with ones who are.

Who do you have in your Group 3?

Action to take:

- Try productive conversations or other strategies to convert Group 3 into Group 1
- Divest or spend less time on relationships that are energy negative
- Set clear boundaries
- Protect your energy and be aware of your own inner dialogue
- Be aware of unsolicited advice and the negative effects it can have
- Advocate for yourself with your medical practitioners and build a team that supports you

That's your three groups — my simplified model to help you understand your situation. Relationships are complicated and there will most likely be people that don't fit neatly into these buckets. Navigating relationships successfully could be a whole book in itself!

One last relationship to end on is the relationship you have with yourself. You are the most important person you need onside for your marathon journey. You need to believe in yourself. Be kind to yourself. Advocate for yourself. Give yourself what you need. Be as gentle as you can to yourself.

On some days, your inner voice may go a bit wild, and you'll struggle to do the above. That's okay — we all have those days. The important thing is you start again the next day, being kind, supportive and responsive to what you need.

One big lesson I take away from my long-term fatigue experience is that when you need help, if you let them, people will be there to catch you. It might just not be the people you expect. It might even be people you don't know yet!

Long term, your goal for your team is to support you as you get back on your feet and find your health again. Short term, you are looking to enjoy your life to the best of your ability.

> **Free downloadable e-book** — Don't forget your bonus resource that provides support for sparking valuable discussions with the important people in your life. This includes scripts and conversation starters that guide you towards developing shared understanding, deeper bonds and mutual support.
> You can find it at: www.sarahvizer.com/tootiredtothink

Putting it into practice

Take some time to consider your current relationships.

1. What could you do to help achieve the golden rule in your life? i.e. *'only do things or have interactions that give you more energy than they require from you.'*
   - What could you **stop** doing?
   - What could you **do less** of?
   - What could you **do more** of?
   - What could you **continue** doing?
   - What could you **start** doing?

2. Consider the relationships you have in each group. How can you focus on keeping your relationships as energy positive as possible?

    - Group 1 — People who want to understand and help (energy neutral and energy positive people)
    - Group 2 — People who leave you alone or disappear completely
    - Group 3 — People who actively set you back (energy negative people)

3. Are there any relationships in Groups 2 or 3 that could become Group 1? What would you need for this to happen?

Emotional Summary

- Dealing with long-term fatigue leads to a rollercoaster of emotions, such as those felt with the grief cycle. You typically cycle through the stages and can even get stuck at a certain stage.

- The five stages of the grief cycle are: denial, anger, bargaining, depression and acceptance. A sixth stage has also been proposed, meaning.

- Your mindset, or frame of mind, are your perceptions and beliefs that shape how you make sense of the world and yourself. Both positive and negative elements are usually present within your mindset.

- Overcoming negative elements of your mindset, your unhelpful thought patterns, can take time and practice.

- The unhelpful thought patterns commonly seen with long-term fatigue include feeling like you 'should' be capable of more, catastrophising, overgeneralising, taking things too personally and comparing.

- Strategies you can use to develop a healing mindset — one where you focus on growth and wellbeing — include positively reframing your circumstances, having productive conversations and examining what's in your control. It's also important to focus on yourself, which you can do by remembering who you are and advocating for yourself.

- Even after working on building your healing mindset, the reality is you will have some dark days ahead. You can be prepared by considering your problem areas (goals) and methods to make things more manageable (strategies).

- Managing the people in your life often involves keeping your relationships energy positive where you have control. The golden rule of energy says we only do things or have interactions that give us more energy than they require from us.

- You will most likely have a range of relationships around you as you navigate long-term fatigue; where possible, you want to keep these relationships energy positive.

Medical Reality... Navigating Cracked Systems

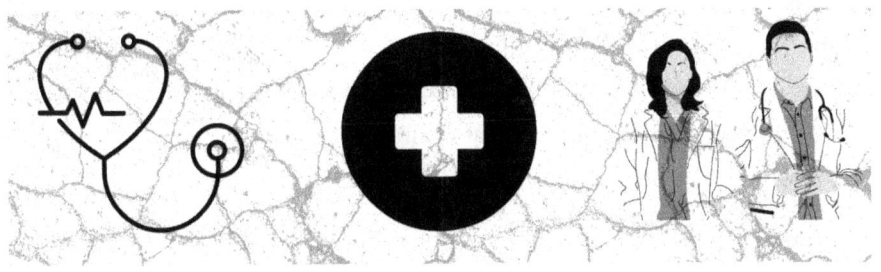

I was exhausted, but I made the appointment anyway. Feelings of cynicism and hope battled it out inside me. I'd been let down so many times in the past by medical practitioners whom I had previously placed on a high pedestal. After fighting fatigue for so many years, those pedestals were no more, and I knew it was a macabre lucky dip of experiences. But this time my luck was in. I found someone who not only had great suggestions but showed genuine empathy for my situation. It's comforting to know there are some true gems out there.

You might be one of the lucky ones, but too many times navigating our various medical systems can be a process that is exhausting at best, soul-destroying at worst.

The stories emerging from those navigating their marathon journey and seeking help with long-term fatigue reveal a wide range of experiences. Some find answers and solutions relatively quickly, while other struggle for years to receive a diagnosis and effective treatment. The persistence required for the latter is painstakingly difficult as they battle exhaustion and all the other symptoms that accompany it.

My experience navigating the medical system here in Australia for my chronic fatigue syndrome diagnosis and treatment was fraught with wrong turns, bad advice (or no advice), expensive solutions that didn't work, being blamed for them not working and a healthy dose of gaslighting to boot! All up, it's been a gruelling process that drained my physical, mental and financial resources at times, and provided little result.

I've also had some great experiences where I felt seen and heard by the practitioner in front of me. I hold on to these positive experiences and remain deeply grateful for the practitioners who worked to restore my faith in the health system. I'm grateful that their help led to my symptoms being now far less severe than they were; I'm in a good state that's become my new normal.

One of the biggest issues is the vague and non-specific nature of long-term fatigue, as well as the lack of set treatment regime. Tired-all-the-time (TATT) symptoms reported by the patient result in the responsibility of the medical practitioner to first make sure it's not a sign of something more serious. Medical practitioners often do this part well — requesting a full range of tests and evaluations. They will then seek answers from the numbers in front of them.

It's when these numbers don't reveal anything wrong that the cracks in the system start to emerge. A commonly reported experience is this... you've been checked over, had your bloods done, and the tests show you are in the 'normal' ranges, your medical practitioner can't see anything wrong, so you have an unexplained suite of symptoms making your life downright impossible.

Depending on the practitioner, they may have suggestions that help. Or they may take you down the grim path of misdiagnosis. Too often we hear about people having their symptoms dismissed. *'You're depressed'* or *'you're just stressed'* or even *'you need to focus on getting more sleep'* can become the so-called diagnosis, leaving exhausted patients feeling at a loss when they are most vulnerable.

The frustration of these experiences only serves to add to the severity of your condition. You are left to jump the rather large cracks in the system at a time when you're already exhausted. You feel dismissed, misunderstood and at times even gaslit into thinking there is nothing wrong with you or it's *'all in your head'*.

These challenges started with ME/CFS and fibromyalgia, which are both notoriously difficult to diagnose. There are no specific tests for these conditions, so a diagnosis is usually made considering a combination of symptoms and by ruling out other medical conditions. Unfortunately, these difficulties have also been mimicked by the experience of so many experiencing long-COVID.

However, it's not all bad news. From the plethora of long-COVID patients, new light has emerged.

- Dedicated long-COVID clinics have popped up around the globe offering treatment and support.

- A multitude of research projects are being conducted around long-COVID and ME/CFS with new information now coming to light.
- Online support groups host large numbers who eagerly share research studies and effective treatment protocols with each other. They also offer valuable emotional support, missing for too long within this community.

We can only live in hope that this will bring a new dawn for diagnosis and treatment of long-term fatigue conditions.

This section is all about understanding what support you need navigating your current medical system.

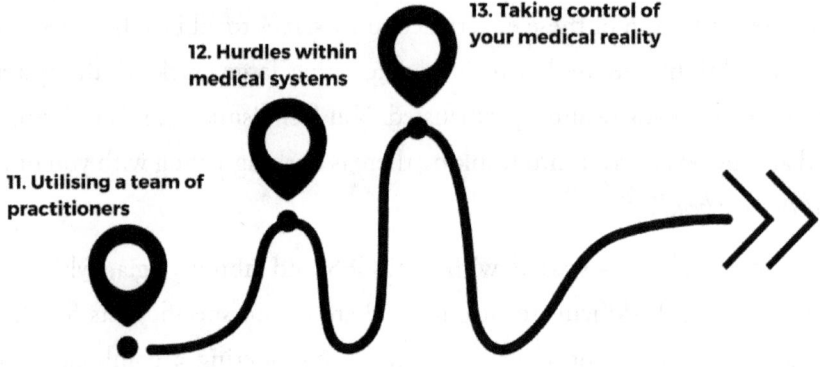

Figure 19 — Medical Reality Chapter Roadmap

- Chapter 11 looks at the range of different practices available and how important it is to take a multidisciplinary approach.
- Chapter 12 assesses the common hurdles that often need to be overcome when looking for support.

- Chapter 13 ends by setting yourself a medical goal — helping you feel informed, prepared and empowered to find the medical support and practitioner team you need to make progress towards feeling better, whatever that looks like for you.

This is your medical reality: where there is little consensus on how long-term fatigue should present and be treated, or even whether it's even a real condition; where a range of treatment options are available to you if you have the patience and perseverance to go find them; where, over time, you can hope to build your team of supportive practitioners who can help you navigate your marathon of improvement and personal recovery, discovering your new normal.

Chapter 11
Utilising a Team of Practitioners

Ava is a 40-year-old management consultant from Atlanta, Georgia. She didn't set out to go doctor shopping, but sadly that is what eventuated. Ava started feeling exhausted and went to her normal doctor. After a diagnosis of anxiety and depression, and taking medication that didn't work, Ava eventually consulted a (very expensive) integrative doctor who diagnosed ME/CFS. Despite the cost, it was a relief to have a proper diagnosis and a pathway for treatment. Ava was prescribed an assortment of natural supplements, as well as psychological support. She was also urged to eat a range of probiotic foods.

After two years, Ava's fatigue was not improving, so she made the decision to move doctors once again. After a series of missteps, she eventually found a local doctor who had researched the ME/CFS condition and was knowledgeable around the latest treatments.

This doctor acted as Ava's primary care contact and referred her to a specialist who prescribed the medication low-dose naltrexone. She was grateful to find that her condition started improving, albeit slowly. Over the following two years, Ava was able to find assistance through a mix of medication, psychological support and consulting with a dietitian. She has now improved to the point that she no longer feels the effects of PEM. She is ready to consult with an exercise physiologist to start the process of exploring how to safely incorporate more movement into her week.

Throughout this section, I will refer to practitioners. There are a lot of different areas that fall under this one umbrella term, used to describe all the different professionals (medical or otherwise) that form part of your treatment team.

You can see from Ava's experience in the snapshot above that she consulted with a wide range of practitioners over the years, including multiple medical doctors, an integrative doctor, a specialist in fatigue, a psychologist, a dietitian and most recently an exercise physiologist.

Chronic conditions such as long-term fatigue usually require a team of practitioners to help with their treatment, particularly at the beginning of their marathon journey. Ava's experience is not atypical — many people with long-term fatigue struggle to find the right team who can diagnose and manage their condition. It can often take time, years even, and can become a huge drain on our time, energy and financial resources.

There are a range of different medical practices you can consult. The following is a quick overview of the different options that may be available in your country.

Conventional/Western medicine/Allopathic medicine — This type of medicine is practiced by professionals who have obtained a medical degree from a recognised medical school and are licensed to practice in their respective countries.

It is a science-based approach that focuses on the physical body, using drugs, surgeries and other medical procedures to treat illness and disease. This approach relies on scientific research and evidence-based medicine to determine safety and effectiveness of medical treatments.

For long-term fatigue, these are your doctors or general practitioners (commonly called GPs) that can act as your **primary care doctor**. They can become your medical central point of contact, referring you to specialists and helping you navigate what other professions would be useful, such as mental health and naturopathic support.

Appointments are most often short, and these doctors are usually not considered a specialist in any field unless they have a particular interest and have undertaken more specific training.

Integrative medicine involves a conventionally trained doctor who has completed more training and are therefore considered more of a specialist. They combine treatments from conventional medicine with alternative or complementary therapies where there is high-quality evidence of safety and effectiveness. They focus on treating the whole person, rather than just the symptoms of the condition, and addressing underlying causes.

For long-term fatigue, an integrative doctor can act as a **specialist**. They will generally cost more than your primary care doctor, but spend more time with you getting to know your condition on a deeper level.

Integrative medicine is not intended to replace conventional medical care, but rather to complement it. An integrative doctor can use a range of therapies, including medication, nutritional supplements, herbal remedies, acupuncture, diet, massage and mindfulness practices.

Functional medicine is also a science-based, holistic approach that integrates conventional medicine with alternate and complementary therapies.

It aims to address the underlying causes of disease and addresses the whole person, not just an isolated set of symptoms.

This medicine emphasises a **patient-centred approach** that aims to get to the root causes of chronic illnesses. It can do this by understanding factors such as your health history, genetic makeup, lifestyle choices and environment.

For long-term fatigue, functional medicine practitioners[29] can work collaboratively with other healthcare professionals, such as your primary care doctor, nutritionists, physical therapists and mental health professionals to provide a comprehensive care plan. Be aware this can involve many different assessments and cost a lot more than general care.

Other traditional medicines

There are also a range of traditional medical practices (may be referred to as **natural medicine**) that will typically work alongside conventional medicine to complement the approach, or in the case of alternative medicine offer a different solution. They consider the person holistically rather than focusing on a named health condition[30].

These approaches are often used to manage symptoms and improve quality of life in people with chronic conditions or illnesses. Areas like lifestyle and diet may supplement the medical focus in order to look for **underlying causes** of ill health.

---

29 The Institute for Functional Medicine (IFM) provides information about what functional medicine is about and you can search for accredited practitioners in your country — www.ifm.org
30 A summary of natural medicine is available at the Australian Traditional Medicine Society under 'modalities' — www.atms.com.au/modalities/

A summary of the focus of these traditional medicines is as follows:

- **Alternative medicine** involves approaches that are used *instead of* conventional approaches. Traditional Chinese Medicine is a good example of what we would classify as alternative medicine.
- **Complementary medicine** is when therapies are used *along with* conventional approaches. An example would be someone undergoing chemotherapy (conventional medicine) getting reflexology and massage before treatments to assist with fatigue and nausea (complementary medicine).
- **Naturopathic medicine or naturopathy** is a holistic system of healing that incorporates a range of treatments and natural therapies, with the underlying belief that your body, given the right support, can heal itself[31]. Treatment may involve nutritional advice, dietary changes, herbal medicines, homeopathy, bodywork or nutritional supplements. Naturopaths will not necessarily utilise all these therapies, but will have a range of therapies they specialise in.

Treatments arising from these different traditional medicine approaches that you might consider for long-term fatigue include:

- Natural products such as herbal remedies and dietary supplements
- Mind-body practices such as meditation, yoga, tai chi and acupuncture
- Complementary therapies such as chiropractic care, massage therapy and acupuncture
- Energy therapies such as reiki and kinesiology

---

[31] WebMD offers a simple and practical guide to naturopathic medicine —www.webmd.com/balance/guide/what-is-naturopathic-medicine

- Nutritional and diet-related advice, and homeopathic remedies

Which types of medical practices have you tried?

As you can see from these descriptions, there are many different types of medical practices that are used to treat chronic conditions.

In Western countries, it is most typical to work with a primary care doctor who is a conventionally trained doctor. They become your central point of contact for all things medically related.

People treating all types of chronic conditions have found great efficacy in supplementing their conventional medical care with treatments from these other traditional medicines.

In general, the other types of medical practices outlined should not be used as a substitute for this conventional medical care, particularly for serious or life-threatening conditions. Rather, they are often used *in conjunction* with conventional medicine to provide a more holistic approach to treatment of long-term fatigue.

Your primary care doctor becomes your central point of contact for all things medically related. Do you have this in place?

By maintaining a strong relationship with your primary care doctor, you can be sure that anything you try is safe and appropriate for your condition. This includes mixing medicine, herbal remedies or supplements to ensure they will not react with each other and become harmful to you. Likewise, you want to know that any treatments or therapies you want to try — such as acupuncture, massage or energy healing — will provide you with a good result and not become detrimental to your condition.

With this relationship in place, it opens the door to trying different therapies. Many people have reported sampling complementary, integrative and functional therapies, and it can pay to keep an open mind around the full spectrum of options you have available to you. You never know what may relieve your symptoms and provide a boost to the energy bank.

I've tried a lot of different therapies over the years with varying success. I'll give you two examples — one therapy that worked and one that didn't.

1. **What didn't work — acupuncture.** I went to a reputable acupuncturist and explained my complete lack of energy resulting from my chronic fatigue syndrome. He was keen to help and placed needles to stimulate my energy system. I paid and left feeling okay. Around three hours later, I suddenly felt a jolt of energy rush through my body and my heart start to race, which felt quite scary. I still had my usual afternoon exhaustion, but could not rest as this 'other' energy was coursing through my body. It was an unpleasant experience and exhausted me even further rather than helping with my fatigue.

2. **What did work — floating.** When nothing else helped my fatigue, I found floating in specially designed sensory deprivation tanks was the only thing that gave me an energy boost. Attracted by the theory that one hour of floating can be more restorative than four to eight hours of deep sleep, I found the mixture of salt and magnesium required no effort from my body or mind, and allowed for my first truly relaxing experience in weeks. It was a much-needed rest and soothed my aching body. The biggest relief came from finding something that was worth the 'investment' of my valuable energy.

These are my experiences only and might not be typical for someone else. I've heard of people with long-COVID having much better success with acupuncture for example. Floating is also not for everyone as it can seem like a weird and wonderful treatment experience all rolled into one!

Sometimes it will come down to the resources you have available. Trying different therapies can become a high cost of energy, time and money and not everyone with long-term fatigue has access to those resources.

The idea is to try a few different suggestions and options, as much as your energy envelope allows, in order to see what will work for you. As long as it's not dangerous to your condition, you never know what will help you. Working with your primary care doctor, you can be in the driver's seat deciding what is best for your situation.

A multidisciplinary approach

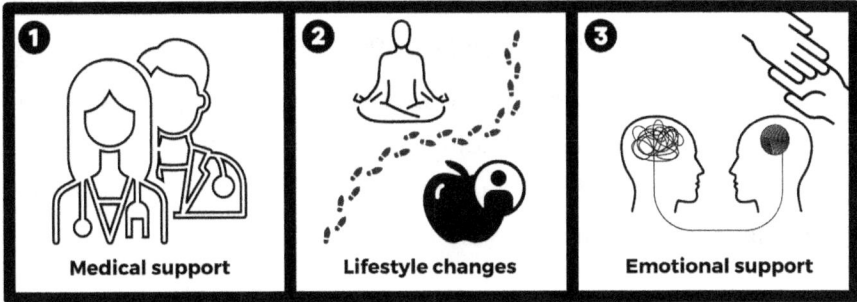

Figure 20 — Elements of a Multidisciplinary Approach

As we have seen, long-term fatigue is a complex condition. Most likely, you will need to deal with range of different practitioners. I refer to this as a multidisciplinary approach and have identified three different areas of support you can access:

1. **Medical support** including working with your primary care doctor and taking medications where applicable
2. **Lifestyle changes** across aspects such as diet and physical activity
3. **Emotional support** for the emotional and psychological impacts

A multidisciplinary approach involves your team of practitioners working together to develop a personalised treatment plan that addresses all the aspects of your condition. This recognises the complex nature of your condition.

1. **For medical support,** we've discussed working with one primary care doctor. This is your central point of contact who will oversee all your care, prescribe medications where applicable and coordinate with other medical practices and specialists. Building a relationship with this doctor is crucial as it will then inform all your other areas of treatment.

   From here, your primary care doctor can refer you to relevant specialists or other services that can assist your condition.

   For long-COVID, specialised clinics have been set up across various countries. Suggestions on finding out what is available to you include: searching online, asking your primary care doctor's recommendation, asking in online forums.

2. **For lifestyle changes,** it is important to work with practitioners who understand your long-term fatigue condition. Some of the disciplines available include the following:

   - **Dieticians or nutritionists** can assist you by identifying any dietary changes that support your overall health and energy levels. I found working with a low-chemical diet helped immensely with brain fog. Other people have reported efficacy in low inflammation or low histamine diets. A qualified professional can help find what works for you.

   - **Naturopathic support** involves a naturopath incorporating assessments into your treatment plan to investigate the cause of symptoms. They can then personalise your plan to treat these symptoms.

This includes a range of therapies such as nutritional advice, dietary changes, herbal and/or nutritional supplements, suggestions on lifestyle modifications, mind-body techniques, bodywork and homeopathy[32].

- **Health coaches** will not give advice, rather support you to take action on the healthy lifestyle behaviour changes you want to put in place. Your health coach will help you set goals and hold you accountable for keeping them. This is a wonderful profession for building more support and accountability into your world, so you can effectively follow the good advice laid out by other practitioners. You will most likely learn a lot more about yourself, as well as transforming unwanted beliefs as part of this process.[33]

  Caution: As a coach myself, it is my opinion that coaching is best undertaken in the later and more consistent stages of your marathon journey, such as when you are at the end of the onwards and upwards trajectory or at your point of new normal. The earlier stages, particularly the messy middle, do not lend themselves as readily to consistency, goal-setting or accountability.

- **Meditation/gentle yoga/breathwork** are all healing modalities that incorporate elements of peace to your mind, body and spirit. The emphasis becomes finding practitioners who can help you reap the benefits without taxing your resources and putting further stress on your body.

- **Exercise physiologists or physical therapists** can assist in the later stages of your marathon journey with physical deconditioning, helping you build strength and endurance back up again.

---

32 Reference: Hechtman, Leah. 2011, *Clinical Naturopathic medicine*, Elsevier Australia
33 The National Board for Health and Wellness Coaching provides a good explanation of what is a health coach and how they can help —nbhwc.org/what-is-a-health-coach/

Caution: *When it comes to movement and exercise with long-term fatigue conditions, there is a growing body of evidence that demonstrates strenuous physical activity, or even trying to exercise at all, is counterproductive at best and harmful at worst when PEM is present.*

*PEM is triggered by exceeding your energy envelope. It can be misconstrued by some experts (including doctors and therapists) as deconditioning, which is the decline of the body's physical function following a period of inactivity, bedrest or a sedentary lifestyle. PEM is **not** deconditioning and should not be treated as such.*

Study upon study has found that physical exertion can make your fatigue symptoms exponentially worse, leading to stress, pain, brain fog, weakness and of course, crushing fatigue.[34] PEM could be considered your safety-indicator that there is a strong biological reason to not push yourself outside of your boundaries. Basically, it's a big flashing warning sign saying, 'Don't go there!' PEM requires pacing and rest in order to be managed.

Over the years, Graded Exercise Therapy (GET) has too often been prescribed as part of the treatment of fatigue conditions by ill-informed practitioners, leading to distress and even worsening of the underlying condition. Even more harmful is that some of us (rightfully) resisting GET are then labelled 'fearful' of activity and advised to seek psychological support, such as CBT to help 'get over it'.

Never be pushed into doing more than what you feel physically capable of doing. The timing of when you seek support from an exercise physiol-

---

34 Various studies such as the one referenced in this article have consistently found that graded exercise therapy almost certainly cause harm for those recovering from ME/CFS. This study found ME/CFS subjects took an average of about two weeks to recover from cardiopulmonary exercise tests, whereas sedentary controls needed only two days. Article link — www.mdpi.com/1648-9144/59/3/571. It is studies such as these that resulted in bodies such as the Centers for Disease Control and Prevention concluding that standard forms of exercise for those with ME/CFS and most recently long-COVID do not help and revising their guidelines for both patients and physicians.

ogist or physical therapist is important, usually most useful when PEM is not present. There is great benefit to working with an experienced therapist, particularly one who understands your condition or is willing to learn. However, only engage when you feel it's the right time for your condition, and you have the energy to invest in this therapy.

- **Dentists** — While not strictly a lifestyle change, dental issues and bad mouth hygiene can cause infection, adding to fatigue and weakening your immune system. You might want to schedule yourself a check-up to look for any issues and ensure you are maintaining good oral health. I chose to remove all old amalgam (silver) fillings, as some were leaking and I wanted to ensure they were not adding to my fatigue.

  Caution: *When getting local anaesthetic at the dentist, some people with long-term fatigue have found the adrenaline can cause a flare-up of symptoms. If this is the case, ask if there are adrenaline-free options.*

3. **For emotional support,** there is a range of practitioners available, including for counselling, psychology and psychiatry. Not only is the long-term, marathon nature of the condition difficult to deal with, but it is commonly accompanied by psychological effects, such as depression, anxiety, or post-traumatic stress disorder (PTSD). A qualified therapist can help manage these conditions, providing coping mechanisms and deeper support.

The goal of a multidisciplinary approach is to use the full spectrum of options available to treat the symptoms and help improve your overall quality of life.

One final note of caution is to carefully select the practitioners you want to work with and who understand your condition. Chapter 13 provides a set of criteria to evaluate the practitioners you meet and find your gems.

Next is a consideration of the hurdles you might face as you put together your practitioner team and navigate your country's medical system.

Putting it into practice

Considering all the various medical practices and practitioner options, use the space below to explore how you can expand your team and take a multidisciplinary approach.

1. Who do you have in your current practitioner team?
2. What have you have tried in the past and what was the outcome?
3. Taking a multidisciplinary approach, what might be beneficial to try in the future?
    a. Medical support
    b. Lifestyle changes
    c. Emotional support

Chapter 12
Hurdles Within Medical Systems

Rachael is an IT sales consultant from Melbourne, Australia. She was 59 when first diagnosed with fibromyalgia. It took her 12 long months to finally receive this diagnosis.

Rachael originally went to her doctor with unexplained pain in her body and growing debilitating fatigue. She woke up every morning feeling stiff and sore, and found even simple tasks like getting dressed or cooking dinner exhausting.

Her primary care doctor ran a series of blood tests, and everything came back within the normal range. Rachael felt emotional about her deteriorating condition and her doctor suggested it might be stress-related. They recommended trying relaxation techniques and including more exercise in her day.

Rachael felt frustrated and dismissed, but resolved to try to relax and exercise more. This just seemed to make things even worse; in particular, exercise was painful and exhausting. After dropping down to part-time work, she eventually returned to the doctor and insisted on a referral to a specialist.

Rachael was not prioritised. After a lengthy five-month wait to see a rheumatologist, she underwent a battery of tests that ruled out other conditions — finally diagnosing fibromyalgia. She could then start treatment with a combination of medication, physical therapy and stress-reduction techniques. By then, Rachael had suffered an entire year of pain and exhaustion with minimal medical assistance.

Rachael felt a mix of anger, anxiety and depression from her experience, which no doubt worsened her fibromyalgia. She felt her primary care doctor had been flippant about her symptoms, so eventually moved to someone more thorough and understanding. She has turned this around and views her experiences as a huge learning curve. She now shares her story as an advocate for fibromyalgia awareness, helping others find an easier pathway to diagnosis.

Have you ever had an experience of feeling dismissed or overlooked within your medical system? If so, you are not alone! Rachael's unfortunate experience finding a diagnosis for fibromyalgia in the snapshot above is not a solitary case of misdiagnosis. It's relatively easy to find commentary from people all around the world experiencing long-term fatigue and feeling misunderstood, neglected or unheard within their current medical reality.

This chapter explores the unfortunate lack of understanding of complex conditions, and the deficiencies present in our current educational and medical systems. It's through understanding the hurdles you may face (or have already) that opens the door to more effective navigation of the medical system and finding practitioners who can help.

My intention is to help you more effectively overcome these hurdles, or at least not be surprised if they happen to you. Ideally, the wisdom contained in this chapter will help circumvent some of the more heartbreaking pain that can unfold:

- Emotional pain from feeling dismissed, unheard, frustrated, anxious and depressed
- Financial pain from feeling like an appointment is wasted or the 'expert' did not understand your condition
- Physical pain when untreated conditions wreak havoc on the body

Based on the stories of hundreds of others who have navigated long-term fatigue, let's look at how five common hurdles unfold.

Common hurdles

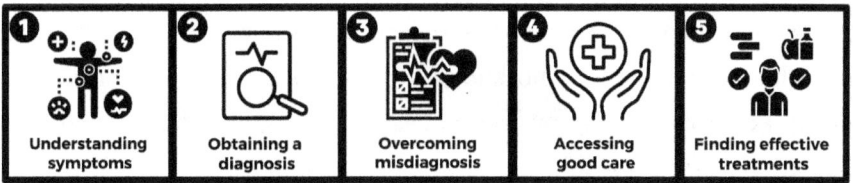

Figure 21 — Common Hurdles Navigating Medical Systems

Hurdle 1 — Understanding your own symptoms.

The common hurdles faced within the management of long-term fatigue start with your own clarity of thought and understanding your symptoms. Untangling your symptoms and accurately describing your day-to-day experience while in a fog of fatigue can feel downright impossible.

Long-term fatigue can originate from any number of different conditions, or even be the condition in itself. It can be difficult for you as the patient to pinpoint what's going on and equally difficult for the practitioner to isolate the symptoms. It's also human nature to fixate on symptoms that are more specific and therefore more easily treated.

With long-COVID, you're often dealing with a complex mix of symptoms. Some might even seem quite bizarre or unexpected such as hair loss, COVID toes (swelling or discolouration) and phantom smells or tastes.

For ME/CFS and fibromyalgia, symptoms can seem vague or build over time. This can include symptoms like a growing tiredness after a big event, problems with bloating, constipation or diarrhoea that comes and goes, and unexplained aches and pains.

These types of symptoms can result in difficulty identifying exactly when they started and what you're dealing with.

Hurdle 2 — Obtaining a diagnosis.

Once you do have a handle on what you're experiencing, the next hurdle is finding a practitioner who knows how to make a diagnosis. Too many medical doctors don't know how to deal with long-term fatigue and there are various reasons for this.

Firstly, it doesn't seem to be a condition that is well-taught within mainstream education systems. This may result in your practitioner not having knowledge of productive ways to diagnose and handle your condition. I've even had a doctor advise me there is no such condition as chronic fatigue syndrome — clearly a lack of awareness and education on his behalf.

The other complicating factor we've discussed are the varied and vague symptoms. There seems to be no clear consensus on what they should be to form a diagnosis, with ME/CFS only diagnosed by ruling out all other possibilities. This can be a nightmare scenario for both yourself trying to explain what is going on and for the medical practitioner trying to decipher what exactly they can help with.

In turn, this can lead to a range of issues — incorrect diagnosis, not feeling heard, feeling dismissed or seeing the appointment as a waste of your precious resources (time, *energy* and money).

Hurdle 3 — Overcoming misdiagnosis.

Another hurdle commonly experienced is misdiagnosis or pushing a psychological diagnosis over a physical condition. Practitioners can attribute fatigue to something that isn't the case at all.

Rather than being a genuine medical condition in its own right, a practitioner may look at fatigue as being due to other factors, such as personal weakness, lack of motivation or psychological issues like untreated anxiety or depression. This can feel like a slap in the face, especially at a time when you're feeling vulnerable. Examples of misdiagnosis often include mental health conditions such as stress, anxiety or depression.

Let's consider depression and how it can become a misdiagnosis. Many people do report feeling depressed when dealing with long-term fatigue. Like the chicken and the egg — is depression causing your feelings of fatigue or might your feelings of depression be a (quite reasonable) reaction to trying to deal with a long-term fatigue condition? Getting help for depression is smart in either case, but not an alternate diagnosis to what is really going on. Ill-informed practitioners can rely on psychological treatments such as CBT, missing the underlying fatigue diagnosis.

Misdiagnosis can also be a failure to recognise the severity of the condition. Some practitioners can downplay fatigue with reports such as '*trouble sleeping*'. This implies an acknowledgment of lethargy, but does not capture the extent to which long-term fatigue can impact your life.

Misdiagnosis can lead to distressing and harmful treatments, such as the suggestion of physical activity. For anyone with long-term fatigue, GET or even just your normal exercise routine is not recommended as it can lead to debilitating PEM, not to mention leaving you feeling even more down when you cannot do what your doctor has prescribed.

Hurdle 4 — Accessing good care.

Finding good practitioner assistance and overcoming misconceptions and bias can become our next hurdle. Depending on your age, gender, ethnicity and other factors, you may encounter practitioners who make broad assumptions around your condition.

Education and training do not always provide practitioners with an adequate understanding of how to treat long-term fatigue, neither as a symptom nor as a condition. This is where the range of patients that a practitioner has been exposed to can assist — a more experienced practitioner will no doubt have come across other long-term fatigue sufferers within their career.

This still is not a guarantee that the practitioner will understand what you are experiencing. Even my trusted primary care doctor pushed me too early to get moving, urging me to consult with an exercise physiologist. I pushed back knowing I was nowhere near ready, but I felt terrible for doing so. I feared being labelled 'resistant'. Internally, I also questioned whether I was just being 'lazy'. Looking back now, I'm so grateful I did push back, knowing the PEM-hell that could have awaited had I acted on the doctor's suggestions. In the last year, I've been able to join a gym (and even use it!) but this had to be done to my own timeline.

It then becomes about their appetite for exploring vague symptoms. Long-term fatigue requires a lot of time and dedication to treat. It can often feel like more trial and error than actual science. With limited time and resources, finding practitioners who are willing to try different things with you and dig deeper to find the underlying cause of your fatigue can be a struggle. Bonus points if your practitioner keeps up with the latest research, with new knowledge and treatments constantly being unearthed.

Related to lack of training is the lack of research and understanding around long-term fatigue as both a symptom and a condition. With the emergence of long-COVID affecting so many people globally, research has stepped up of late, but at the time of writing there is no one treatment or drug that can be prescribed for any long-term fatigue condition.

And lastly, depending on your location and other factors, it can be difficult to access appropriate care. Issues that regularly occur include long wait times, limited availability of specialists and diagnostic tests, and the cost of treatments. Financial resources can be particularly challenging when dealing with such a long-term condition, particularly if you are not able to work, are not covered by insurance or not able to receive some type of disability payment.

Hurdle 5 — Finding effective treatments to manage symptoms.
Once you've landed on a diagnosis, what do you do when there is no magic bullet? One of the most frustrating aspects of navigating the medical world is a lack of effective treatments available for dealing with long-term fatigue.

In fact, there is no known 'cure', no one treatment or drug protocol to treat the condition quickly and effectively[35]. It can take years and is most often the case that your practitioner team's focus will be on addressing the symptoms.

Many 'treatments' can even feel insulting, such as being referred to a psychologist or even being told to get more exercise (which, as I've mentioned, is not recommended with the existence of PEM). Treatments are usually around managing symptoms rather than trying to find a cure. Sometimes the message is about finding a way to live with your symptoms.

---

35 Various bodies, including the Centers for Disease Control and Prevention have outright stated there is no cure or approved treatment for ME/CFS. Instead, they advise that relief can be provided by treating or managing some symptoms.

When you do try treatments, results will also vary. What works for one person is not guaranteed to work for someone else. We often try multiple treatments at once. In that case, if improvement occurs, you will not be able to pinpoint exactly *what* worked. It may be that these treatments are working in conjunction with each other or just one is effective.

This can be enormously frustrating for the person with the condition. I can only imagine this is frustrating for the practitioner as well. Practitioners who got into the profession to help people can become frustrated with this lack of progress. They can fixate on the minor, more tangible symptoms they know what to do with, such as trying to fix your sleep issues. They may even give up altogether. In extreme cases, there are even examples of practitioners blaming the patient for their lack of progress. This is a particularly cruel form of gaslighting — kicking people when they are already down.

While there is no one treatment, we can hope for signs of improvement in symptoms over time. There have also been many examples where people have made a complete recovery. Hope, indeed.

What hurdles have you experienced?

All in all, dealing with long-term fatigue within chronic conditions can be a marathon event that is both frustrating and debilitating. Unfortunately for too many of us, it's hit or miss as to whether we'll visit a practitioner and find the help we need. Dealing with these cracked medical systems can be a tremendous drain on our already meagre energy, as well as our time and financial resources.

However, it's not all doom and gloom! Our next chapter will explore what you can do to overcome these hurdles and find the help you both need and deserve.

Putting it into practice

Take some time to identify your own experiences with practitioners and within your medical system. Make a quick inventory of any or all the hurdles that you feel you're currently facing.

- Hurdle 1 — Understanding your own symptoms
- Hurdle 2 — Obtaining a diagnosis
- Hurdle 3 — Overcoming misdiagnosis
- Hurdle 4 — Accessing good care
- Hurdle 5 — Finding effective treatments to manage symptoms

Chapter 13

Taking Control of your Medical Reality

Amir is 28 and living in Tel Aviv. In March 2021, he contracted COVID-19 and felt ill over several weeks. After recovering from the initial infection, he experienced a range of debilitating symptoms including fatigue, brain fog, shortness of breath and muscle pain.

He visited numerous doctors and specialists over the next few months and was eventually diagnosed with long-COVID. The doctors were sympathetic, but struggled with the unique challenges that long-COVID brings.

Feeling frustrated, Amir stumbled upon a support group for people with long-COVID and met others going through similar experiences. His goal became finding someone who could actually help him, with his biggest breakthrough coming when he heard about a doctor specialising in treating long-COVID patients.

Amir booked an appointment and travelled a long way to meet with this doctor, desperately hoping it was worth his time and energy expen-

diture. It was a relief to find that his support group's recommendation was good — this doctor was worth the effort, and knowledgeable about the latest research and treatments. After reviewing his symptoms and medical history, and completing a series of tests, this doctor was able to develop a treatment plan that has helped Amir. This involved a mix of medication, physical therapy to help with mobility, meditation and breathwork.

Amir has been on a much better path after this and recognises that this one doctor has been a massive turning point in his whole experience. He even has enough mental resources to get back into gaming, a favourite pastime that restores valuable social connection. He has since shared this doctor's recommendations back in the online support group for others to benefit.

Now you've had a chance to consider the hurdles of dealing with your long-term fatigue condition so far, the question becomes what you can do about them.

Amir in the snapshot above had just one goal — to find someone who could help with his long-COVID condition. After months of searching, receiving a recommendation from an online group paid off and the recommended doctor was able to develop a treatment plan that worked — happy days!

We have discussed many times that long-term fatigue conditions are complex. When it comes to finding assistance and overcoming hurdles, it provides clarity to **start with a clear goal around your medical care.** One suggestion for your goal could be something like the following:

*To feel as **informed, prepared and empowered as possible** so that I can take control of my health, gaining effective and positive outcomes for the resources I expend — time, money and energy.*

> This involves **building a team of practitioners** covering both the physical and emotional aspects of dealing with long-term fatigue. This team is knowledgeable on how to diagnose and treat the condition and supports me for however long it takes to find improvement and manage my symptoms.

There are two aspects in the above example (which is more like a *recommendation* from me!) Those two aspects are: feeling informed, prepared and empowered and building a team of helpful practitioners. Let's look at each part in turn.

Tips for feeling informed, prepared and empowered

Tips for building a team of gems

Figure 22 — 2 Elements in Building your Medical Care

Feeling informed, prepared and empowered

This is about approaching your appointments feeling as informed and prepared as possible. In turn, this helps you feel empowered when navigating your medical system — to boldly reject what doesn't feel right and isn't working, and to keep seeking what you do require.

Being informed and prepared **is not** asking you to…

…step into the shoes of your medical practitioners and come up with your own diagnosis.

...turn to Doctor Google or seek advice and remedies from unsubstantiated sources.

Rather **it is** asking you to...

...seek a wide range of informed opinions.

...understand your symptoms well enough so you can explain them with clarity.

...feel confident questioning a diagnosis or treatment when it doesn't feel right or doesn't lead to a good outcome.

...seek second opinions when required.

Doing this allows you to be in the driver's seat of your own medical journey. Navigating a long-term, complex condition requires this of you.

This aspect is about focusing your precious resources in a way that provides the most value for you. These resources include your time, your money and (maybe most importantly) your energy. All three of these resources can be scarce when dealing with long-term, complex conditions.

Your time and money are obviously important, but remember that your energy becomes your most valuable currency. In Chapter 4, we quantified finite energy using the spoon theory and energy units. For someone with limited energy to attend an appointment and travel to and from the location, this alone can use up their full allocation of energy for the whole day!

If a pattern of unproductive appointments emerges, you could be justified in feeling it becomes a waste of your precious energy resources. Not only is there an opportunity cost of what else you could do with your day, but you also face the likelihood of experiencing PEM. Then there's the emotional load that also comes from attending appointments with negative outcomes to consider — even more of an energy drain.

Particularly in times of low energy and fatigue, it is important to find ways to maximise the chance of your appointments going well. This involves getting the most benefit you can in return for your energy expenditure.

Top tips for feeling informed, prepared and empowered

Here are six tips for being as informed, prepared and empowered as possible when attending appointments and meeting with practitioners.

Tip 1: Keep a symptom diary — Fatigue symptoms such as exhaustion and brain fog do not enable you to communicate at your best. Keeping a diary of details around what symptoms you are experiencing will help you provide the best information possible.

Your diary can include details such as:

- Details of the symptom.
- When it occurs.
- How long it lasts for.
- What you were doing at the time e.g. what you were eating, activity you were performing, location that it occurred.
- What factors make it better or worse.

Tip 2: Prepare your own research — Not advising you to turn to Doctor Google, but being as prepared as possible with your own research before your appointment helps you feel more confident and ask more informed questions.

You might be able to find information about your condition for yourself, or recruit someone else to help you with this. There are various organisations that having mailing lists and share relevant information. If you are part of any online support groups, you might find they actively share the latest treatments, journal articles and expert recommendations.

Having this information helps you assess the thoroughness and competence of the person in front of you. You may be better able to interpret their responses. It can also help open the pathways of thinking to consider multiple treatment options for your condition.

This potentially works best when you've been navigating your fatigue condition for a while or you have something definite to research (such as post-viral fatigue or being part of a ME/CFS, fibromyalgia or long-COVID group).

Tip 3 — Challenge the diagnosis — When someone gives you a diagnosis of ABC and you disagree, try a subtle challenge which helps them think in alternative ways.

Examples include:

- *"It could be ABC, but what would be an alternate/different diagnosis?"*
- *"I've heard that XYZ is also a possibility. Can we also consider this?"*

Caution: *You need to have good sources of reference or run the risk of being dismissed.*

Tip 4: Track your lifestyle and habits — Similar to a symptom diary, keeping track of lifestyle habits provides your practitioner with solid information with which to diagnose and treat your condition.

Your tracking can include:

- When and how long you sleep.

- When and what you eat.
- Daily physical activity.
- How you feel during and after that movement.
- Energy levels throughout the day.
- Stress levels throughout the day. (Check in regularly and rate yourself out of 10 for the stress you are feeling.)

One benefit of this information is it can help shut down any leaps in diagnosis, such as: *'you're just stressed'* or *'you need to focus on your diet and physical activity'*.

Tip 5: Prepare a list of medications and supplements — Making a list, including dosage and frequency, assists you to remember the details. It can also help your primary care doctor identify possible interactions or side effects that may cause or add to your fatigue.

Tip 6: Track your progress — Take control of your situation by tracking your progress. This includes taking notes on any changes in your symptoms and the effectiveness of what you've been prescribed. This will make future appointments more productive as you can lead with facts.

These six tips are geared towards helping you overcome the hurdles and find the support you need (and deserve) for your condition. Using these tips, the question now turns to the 'how'. How can you best feel informed, prepared and empowered when navigating your medical system? How can you get the most benefit from the resources expended (time, money and energy) for each appointment you attend?

Part of achieving this is to put together a strong team of practitioners who provide solid support — the next discussion point.

Building a team of gems

You're now as prepared and informed as possible, and feeling empowered. Next, it's time to consider how you can build a team of the best possible practitioners for your situation.

I really want to acknowledge the many wonderful practitioners who are dedicated to helping their patients, and will show kindness and compassion for your condition. The best of these recognise that this is a complex condition, can help by providing an accurate diagnosis, and will provide suggestions on how to treat your fatigue and other symptoms. Let's call them **our gems.**

The hallmarks of true gems are as follows:

- They listen to you without judgement or being dismissive.
- They demonstrate understanding and belief in your symptoms and condition.
- They actively provide support for what you need.
- They keep up with the latest research and treatment for your condition.
- They are willing to try different treatments, some with varying success.
- They show commitment to supporting you in the long-term rather than looking for a quick fix.

Every time I find a gem, I'm always extremely grateful. I book appointments with them regularly to keep myself front of mind. I make sure they know I'm open to trying different treatments and want them to keep up with the latest research. I also make sure they know how much I appreciate them.

Unfortunately, for every gem I've found, there were also **rocks.** Rocks by my definition are practitioners who at best have not been able to help me.

At worst, they weigh me down, even actively set me back in some way, such as being dismissive or uneducated around long-term fatigue.

At face value, it can be frustrating for a medical community that wants to enable you with a diagnosis and to feel like they are making a difference to your health. The reality is that long-term fatigue is frustratingly difficult to explain, let alone resolve.

I suspect there is ego involved with some of the rocks, where the practitioner can gaslight you into thinking your symptoms are not real or should be resolving within a certain timeframe. The implication here is dangerous: that you are not trying; that you are untreatable; that you are not following protocol; that you are failing.

There is no standard timeline for resolving long-term fatigue and any expectation put upon you can be downright harmful at a time when you are already feeling fatigued.

Confusingly, I've also had practitioners who are both gems and rocks. The gem part is they have some suggestions that are useful. The rock? Their attitude can be dismissive, reek of *you should be better by now* after trying a few things, or under-reporting the real seriousness of my condition.

Just like fossicking, you want to sift through — keeping the gems and where possible ditching the rocks!

Sometimes dealing with the rocks is unavoidable, for example, when they're a specialist. In these cases, hopefully, you can gather enough other gems on your team to ensure you are receiving good advice and can tolerate the odd lapse in bad manners or lack of emotional intelligence!

To support your multidisciplinary approach, your team of gems covers the physical and emotional aspects of dealing with long-term fatigue. This includes practitioners across medical support, lifestyle changes and emotional support.

We noted that your multidisciplinary team is led by one primary care doctor as a central point of contact — your most important gem! From here, you can work together to develop a personalised treatment plan. This will address all the aspects of your condition and help you build your team of gems that forms your full treatment team.

Top tips for building a team of gems.
Here are six tips for building the supportive team of practitioners, your team of gems, that is needed to navigate a long-term and complex fatigue condition.

Tip 1: Find a primary care doctor — As a first priority, find a doctor who is local to you and you consider to be a gem. You need to trust and feel comfortable with this person as you will build a long-term relationship with them. They will be your central point of contact to oversee your care, prescribe medications where applicable and coordinate with other practitioners and specialists.

Tip 2: Ask for recommendations from others with your condition — Finding local people to ask can be an issue, but you can now seek advice from a range of sources through online groups. The benefit of obtaining a recommendation is you have a better understanding of the practitioner and a greater chance of not wasting your time, money and energy resources at the appointment.

Tip 3: Evaluate each practitioner — You want to ensure each practitioner is a true gem and able to help you. To assess whether they are suitable, some questions you could ask include:

1. **Competence around your condition** — Have you treated patients with long-term fatigue before?

2. **Tolerance for ambiguity** — How would you treat complex conditions with unclear symptoms?
3. **Patience to last the distance** — How long on average does it take to find a treatment that works for long-term fatigue?
4. **Keeping up with the latest information** — Have you read any recent research around long-term fatigue that could be relevant to my situation?

Tip 4: Advocate for yourself — We might be tempted to put doctors or specialists on a knowledge pedestal. The reality is like any profession — there are good and bad practitioners. There are also practitioners who are a good fit for you, as well as ones who are not. If you feel your concerns are not being heard or taken seriously, or are being dismissed, then empower yourself to speak up and advocate for yourself. You can always ask for more information or a second opinion.

Tip 5: Change practitioners — In some cases, trying to change the mind of a practitioner even if they have been in your life for years is most likely wasted effort. A better use of your limited resources is to move on. Find the team that has the know-how and willingness to support you. Know there are medical practitioners who do read up about your condition and will understand what you are going through.

Tip 6: Take a trusted contact with you — Taking someone along to appointments can assist you in understanding the information being presented. They can also provide confidence and a boost when it comes to advocating for yourself.

Caution: When taking someone with you, choose this person with care and make sure they have a clear role description that they stick to in the appointment. Having too many people in an appointment can make it even more exhausting.

You also need to be careful of this person taking over the appointment or adding another point of view, which can confuse the issue.

How can you best put together your team of gems?
These six tips are geared towards helping you put together the best team of practitioners possible to help you diagnose and manage your condition.

As the fairy tale goes, the sad truth is you might need to kiss a few frogs before you find your prince / princess - your true gems. When you're critically lacking in energy, this can seem like a big mountain to climb.

The most important role in your team is your primary care doctor. Your marathon journey of finding new practitioners and attending appointments can all be exhausting. With a primary care doctor in place, you can at least be assured you have a solid base of medical care to build off and can create your team over time with their support.

Putting it into practice
Take a bit of time now to bring it all together — building your team and planning how you may achieve your medical goal. You can start with the following:

- **Your team** — Who is your primary care contact and wider team of practitioners? If you don't yet have in place a local primary care doctor that you trust, then this is the first action to take.
- **Current hurdles** — A quick summary of any or all the hurdles that you feel you're currently facing.
- **Goal relating to medical choices** — Write down in your own words the goal you want to set for your medical care around your long-term fatigue. You might borrow the wording of the example in this section or decide on your own goal.

- **Actions to take** — What are the immediate actions you want to take to achieve your goal, feel informed, supported and empowered and build your team of gems? A massive list of actions can become overwhelming, so I suggest you focus on the top two or three that will make the most difference.

For example: *Find a new primary care contact within 5km of my house within four weeks. To do this, I will seek local recommendations and attend one appointment a week until I find someone I trust.*

Medical Summary

- Being long-term and complex, diagnosing and managing conditions within the sphere of long-term fatigue requires a team of practitioners. This involves taking a multidisciplinary approach and covers medical support, lifestyle changes and emotional support.

- Building a trusting and open relationship with your primary care doctor is a crucial first step. In turn, that person acts as your central point of contact for all things medically related — overseeing your care, prescribing medications where applicable and coordinating other medical practices and specialists.

- Common hurdles you might face in your medical system include: understanding your own symptoms; obtaining a diagnosis; overcoming misdiagnosis; accessing good care; finding effective treatments to manage your symptoms.

- Overcoming these hurdles starts with setting a clear goal for your medical care. There are two aspects to any goal you set around your medical choices: Feeling informed, prepared and empowered and putting together your team of practitioners, your team of gems.

- Feeling informed, prepared and empowered will not only help you better navigate your country's medical system, but also help you get the most benefit from the resources expended for each appointment you attend. Resources include your time, your finances and (most importantly) your energy.

- Your team of gems includes practitioners dedicated to helping you manage your condition, assist with an accurate diagnosis and identify up-to-date treatments. They are willing to support you in the long term. The idea is to sift through, keeping the gems and where possible ditching the rocks!

Getting the Help you Need...What Works and What Doesn't

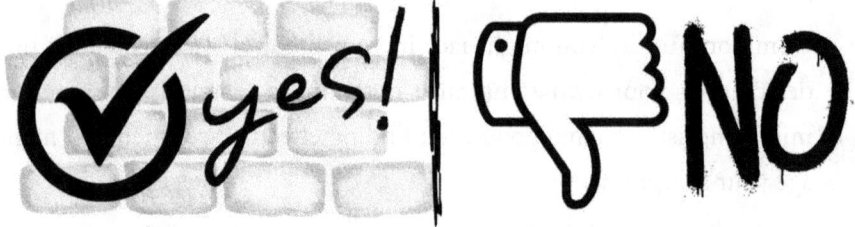

This is where the rubber hits the road — getting you the help you need to navigate your marathon journey.

Unfortunately, we've seen how treatment of this condition can be hit or miss, as there is no set of standardised treatments that all doctors will prescribe. With a growing focus on research around fatigue, particularly long-COVID, there is hope of change and more standardised treatments to come. Until then, it can become a process of building the support structures you need brick by brick based on what works for you.

This section will focus on the factors that do not change. These are the big-picture focus areas that underpin how you approach treating your condition. It will give you a taste of what works and (perhaps even more importantly) what doesn't as you navigate your condition.

To date, I've not found the 'magic bullet' that provides the instant fix we all want so badly. Gradually over time, you'll be able to unpick the layers in this guide. With chronic conditions, it's usually not just one thing that leads to improvement, rather a range of different interventions that eventually bear fruit.

I've felt a gradual lifting of brain fog, a partial restoration of energy. Yet when I overdo it, I'm right back to experiencing the symptom over again, at least temporarily. For me, it's not about never experiencing a crash again, rather my results are around how quickly I can recover. Over time, my ability to rebound strengthens and it takes me less time to return to a baseline level of energy.

I've found these types of results can be difficult to notice at first, especially if I'm not paying attention. It can be disheartening when you don't see results straight away, so easy to try something once and conclude it's not working. Just because you can't measure improvement immediately, it doesn't mean there's no benefit. You wouldn't go to the gym a handful of times and expect a six-pack result, or eat healthily for a day and expect to lose weight!

In the same way, results can be gradual, but lead to long-term improvements over time. Your healing mindset allows you this time to experiment. The challenge is keeping perspective when experimenting with different strategies, particularly when you're operating with such limited energy resources. Your changes may also be quite substantial, even requiring a change in lifestyle. This takes time and patience to not only implement, but also embed.

Implementing these helpful actions and finding your balance is not meant to be a burden. My advice is to start small. To avoid overload, it's okay to try just one action at a time. When you have limited energy, you can pick a chapter that speaks to you, or even get someone else to read it for you and make suggestions. Obviously, they need to be someone you trust (and like), or this can become a whole new recipe for pain!

You will find this section highly practical, providing many opportunities for reflection. Keep your pen and notebook handy, or your computer close, so you can record your own observations and lessons.

This section starts with the basic lifestyle factors that are within your control and help with overall fatigue management. These are the bricks in your foundation, the tried-and-true measures that help you reach your levels of improvement and personal recovery, discovering your new normal.

Let's get started!

Note: If you have skipped straight to the help section, here is a reminder of what two of the commonly used acronyms from Chapter 2 stand for:

PEM — PEM stands for post-exertional malaise. It is what you're feeling when you do too much one day and feel like you've been hit by a truck the next! These are the after-effects of physical, mental or emotional exertion. PEM can be triggered by even minor exertion, such as getting up and having a shower, taking a walk, attending a social event, working on your computer or engaging in an emotionally charged conversation. The effects can last for hours, days or even weeks at a time.

POTS — POTS stands for postural orthostatic tachycardia syndrome. It is when your heart races, you feel dizzy or weak, you might shake or sweat with even the slightest of exertion. It can be triggered by as little as walking up a set of stairs and other factors such as dehydration, prolonged bed rest and certain medications. This is a serious medical condition, and it is always important to seek medical assistance for it.

Chapter 14

Lifestyle, Back to Basics

"My wellness journey has had so many twists and turns, but one thing I've found consistently works is eating to a certain rhythm during the day. I find if I get too hungry, I feel weak and dizzy, so I keep nuts and fruit handy for a quick pick-me-up. I try to eat smaller meals more often with only a light meal at night. This helps me get a better quality of sleep — less vivid dreams and not waking up as much. I also stay away from certain additives, especially MSG (flavour enhancer 621), as it tends to give me an instant headache. I've found these changes easy to make overall and the benefit they bring has been incredible for keeping my energy balanced."

— Martine, 54, Sweden

Lifestyle basics is a topic that everyone can benefit from — the basic lifestyle building blocks that work *for* your health, not against it. When you're dealing with long-term fatigue, getting these organised becomes even more important!

After you have all your basic health checks in place, the next step is to work with your primary care doctor to widen your care. Part of this will be focusing on the basic lifestyle factors that aid recovery.

This becomes about you and your lifestyle — making positive changes aimed at you becoming healthier and happier overall.

Covered here are four core lifestyle basics[36], all within your control:

1. Nutrition and hydration
2. Sleeping patterns
3. Stress levels
4. Dealing with POTS

1. **Nutrition and hydration**

When you're tried, stressed, overwhelmed or anxious, eating a healthy diet can go by the wayside. The daily exhaustion present with fatigue can also lead to real difficulty with tasks such as grocery shopping, preparing healthy food and cooking meals in advance.

This can easily result in slipping into bad eating habits that add to our fatigue levels and overall load.

- This can be **physical** by not getting enough nutrition or eating in a way that adds to your energy depletion.
- It can also be **emotional** through judgements or guilt when you're not eating as you'd like to, adding to your mental load.

---

[36] Exercise is another great lifestyle basic, but this can be tricky with long-term fatigue so we will dedicate a whole section to this topic in Chapter 16.

The first challenge becomes finding ways to eat a healthy, balanced diet and drink enough water each day. Good advice usually advocates drinking between 2 and 3 litres of water each day, and including fruits, vegetables, whole grains, healthy fats and lean protein in your daily meals, while avoiding processed, fried, salty and sugary foods. With physical activity drastically reduced in many cases, what we eat also becomes key to trying to maintain a healthy weight.

You can start simply by focusing on this area of life and making it a priority for a while until it becomes a well-worn habit. Strategies to consider include: writing lists to increase your organisation, always having a water bottle handy, taking shortcuts like meal services, getting groceries delivered, asking for help, bulk cooking… Whatever you can do goes a long way to easing the physical and emotional effects that bad eating brings to your condition.

In terms of what we eat, no specific diet has been shown to reduce the symptoms of long-term fatigue in everyone, but a Mediterranean style of eating has been shown to contain a lot of health benefits. There is evidence that some foods may increase symptoms such as brain fog, painful joints and fatigue. Examples of these include high FODMAP foods, or foods containing gluten, food additives or food chemicals, like aspartame and MSG.

Some people, particularly those with long-COVID, have found efficacy with a low histamine diet. Others follow an anti-inflammatory diet. I went through a process with a dietician to test a low-chemical diet — looking at my tolerance to naturally occurring chemicals in foods.

It can be a case of testing different foods to see what helps and what worsens your symptoms. Many people have found they become more sensitive to different foods and other chemicals as time goes on. I found a range of food that no longer suited me, because it added to fatigue. Interestingly, I also developed a range of other skin sensitivities, including sensitivity to makeup and moisturisers that previously caused no reaction. I'd put these on my skin and instantly feel fatigued.

For those of us who get dizzy or have POTS, eating smaller meals more regularly can help ease these symptoms. I get to a 'critical' low-energy state when I'm hungry, so I've learnt that eating protein-rich meals earlier in the day helps stabilise my energy throughout the afternoon and evening.

You may need supplements to your diet to correct any nutrient imbalances. Working with your primary care doctor, you can find professionals to evaluate your needs. There are no set recommendations on what supplements work best for treating long-term fatigue, but specialists such as integrative doctors[37] will usually try a range.

Your long game here is to feed your body what it needs to feel less fatigue and other symptoms, and gain more energy. I know for sure that my body gives me feedback on what's good for me to consume long term. I feel it — in the clarity of my thoughts, in my energy levels, in my mood. Consulting first with your doctor and then with a professional such as a nutritionist or dietician reveals the best way for you to eat right now considering your own unique situation.

2. Sleeping patterns

Next, let's tackle how to get a good night's sleep. Your body heals and regenerates during sleep, so getting seven to nine hours (or more) of sleep per night remains one of the most important considerations with any health condition, particularly long-term fatigue. You need at least four hours of uninterrupted sleep to get into your restorative phase of sleep[38].

---

37   Refer to the Medical Reality section, particularly Chapter 11 — utilising a team of practitioners — to find out what types of medical support you have available to you in addition to your primary care doctor.
38   COVID care group article by Delainne Bond is an informative resource for brain fog, including a section on what you can do to help and information on sleep. Article link — www.covidcaregroup.org/blog/covid-brain-fog

This is what is generally recommended. However, with long-term fatigue conditions, there are many ways that sleep might be playing out for you.

1. You may already be getting good sleep at night.
2. You may be in a pattern of sleeping a lot during the day then not being able to sleep at night.
3. You might be getting lots of sleep, but it's still not enough to wake up feeling refreshed.

All these scenarios are quite typical and most likely you are already doing a lot of sleeping (or just resting) to manage your fatigue. General advice you will most likely be given by professionals in terms of rest is to listen to what your body needs. Long-term fatigue isn't necessarily something that can be fixed with a good night's sleep, but getting enough quality sleep can help over time. It also helps emotionally — being awake all night can be boring and lonely!

The first step is to address any symptoms that inhibit your sleep, such as pain or discomfort. Fibromyalgia can be particularly painful and long-COVID also comes with a vast array of symptoms that can inhibit sleep. Fibromyalgia might require improvement in your serotonin levels[39]. Working with your medical team, you can prioritise getting them under control, such as taking pain medication or looking for underlying conditions such as sleep apnoea.

The next step is to establish a relaxing bedtime routine. The end of this section provides a simple evidence-based bedtime routine. From reading in depth about this subject, the general advice I've seen appears consistent —

---

39 Dr Brady's work in his book *The Fibro Fix* looks at gut issues in fibromyalgia and how to restore/improve any serotonin imbalances.

not to lie awake indefinitely. If you're not asleep in 20 minutes, then get up and do something relaxing, like reading a book until you're ready to sleep. Where possible, limit blue light sources, using red night lights for vision instead. You can use amber light bulbs in your home for a softer light. Blue light blocking glasses can help minimise the blue effects when looking at screens or watching TV. There is also software that adapts your computer's screen brightness to the time of day.

Just a note about sunlight. This helps us wake up naturally and feel more alert. It also helps regulate our circadian rhythms (internal body clock), having a flow-on effect for the rest of the day and helping us better sleep at night. So, get your daily dose of natural sunlight or bright light. Open your blinds first thing in the morning and enjoy that light! If you can't get outside, it might be worthwhile researching lamps available to you that mimic natural sunlight.

Another common issue is having an anxious, busy, worrying mind. If you do, try a good old-fashioned brain dump before you go to bed. This involves writing down anything and everything that's on your mind to get it out of your head. With no technology, having a journal beside your bed is a good method of doing this. This is also good if you're awake at 2am with a head buzzing with thoughts — just have another brain dump.

Finally, if you're having bad sleep at night, bring this up with your primary care doctor. They may prescribe a sleeping aid and can hopefully help ease other issues such as pain. They may also help you try natural supplements or the hormone melatonin that has properties that aid sleep. Your primary care doctor is there to help find the support you need and test for adverse reactions.

The following is a simple and relaxing bedtime routine that will maximise your chances of getting enough sleep each night. I've developed this routine over time from various sources. It contains general advice only that is recommended by health practitioners and is not specific for any condition.

During the day

- **Sunlight** — Try for 30 minutes of sunlight exposure each day, particularly morning sun. If you can't get outside, it might be worthwhile researching lamps available to you that mimic natural sunlight.
- **Stimulants** — Avoid what you know will interrupt your sleep — typically things like alcohol and nicotine. Caffeine in the afternoon or evening also dramatically affects some people's sleep activity.
- **Physical activity** — Keep workouts or physical activity at least two to three hours before bedtime.
- **Eating and drinking** — Stop eating and drinking lots of liquids two to three hours before bedtime.
- **Bed for sleep** — You want to associate your bed with sleeping, so no eating or working.

Getting ready for bed

- **Calming activities** — Instead of screens, what do you enjoy doing that calms down your mind and body? This might be a shower or bath, gentle yoga, reading a book, listening to music or a podcast, deep breathing, mindful time or meditation or any other feel-good activity.
- **Bedtime consistency** — Stick to a consistent sleep schedule, including when you start your wind down and bedtime.
- **Limit screen time** — Electronics like computers, phones and televisions emit blue light and restrain the production of melatonin, a hormone important for sleep. Turn these off an hour before bedtime.

- **Limit blue light sources** — Where possible, block out blue light sources from your home lighting and electronics, and replace with red light instead. You can use amber light bulbs in your home for a softer light. Blue light blocking glasses can help minimise the blue effects when looking at screens or watching TV. There is also software that adapts your computer's screen brightness to the time of day.
- **Brain dump** — When you have a lot on your mind, use a journal or notebook to clear your mind. This is especially helpful if you tend to worry, stress or ruminate.
- **Dim the lights** — This will help you know it's time for sleep.

Going to sleep

- **Room temperature** — Keep your room cool and comfortable for better sleep.
- **Room darkness** — Keep your room as dark as possible with blinds, curtains or an eye mask.
- **Electronics** — Keep your phone or other electronics away from you or in another room. Remember good old-fashioned alarm clocks!
- **Diffuse lavender** — You may find this helpful in reducing anxiety.
- **White noise** — Ambient noise like a relaxing meditation track or a fan can help you relax.
- **Deep breathing** — This activates your relaxation response, so if you wake up in the night try a few deep breaths.

This simple, evidence-based routine might seem like a lot to take in, and I'd urge you to start with just one or two tweaks to your current practices to begin with, gradually adding to this over time.

When I was at the peak of my fatigue and sleep was so important, I focused on just the smallest of things — filling my room with beautiful scents, only drinking one cup of coffee in the morning to limit caffeine intake, keeping my blinds and windows open to make sure I had plenty of fresh air, and sitting with my pups for 10 minutes in the morning sunlight (drinking that coffee!).

As my energy gradually improved, I started adding in more good practices — using the brain dump method in my journal (particularly at 3am!), napping in places other than my bedroom to keep my bed for sleeping at night and listening to podcasts that required little energy before sleep instead of being on screens.

Step by step, slowly improving my sleep practices has been one of the best methods I know to support my improvement in fatigue levels. On the flip side, not having good sleep practices in place can add to both the physical and mental stress in your life. Luckily this is the next topic!

3. **Stress levels**

Living with long-term fatigue can be highly stressful. Never a truer statement has been made! Stress might be an underlying precursor that has contributed to your initial condition, or it might arise during the management of your condition. No matter what, it is a sure-fire way to bring about further fatigue.

Stress is often described as feeling overloaded, wound-up, tense, worried. It's most likely to be when you feel you can't cope, or you feel under threat or some type of conflict, even if that means conflict within yourself.

In controlled amounts, stress allows you to improve your performance. However, when prolonged, stress can contribute to serious health issues as well as exacerbate your already serious fatigue condition.

Stress is a biological response that forms a natural part of your body's defence system. This response is a balance between two states. **Fight, flight or freeze** activates your **sympathetic nervous system** and energises your body ready to react. **Rest and digest** activates your **parasympathetic nervous system** and calms everything down, important for functions like growth, storing energy in your body and digesting your latest meal.

Under threat or under stress, your fight, flight or freeze response is activated, flooding your system with stress hormones such as adrenaline and cortisol. When you need to kick into action, this stress response is appropriate as it provides an energy release and blood flowing to your muscles for speed. This response is designed to last around 90 seconds, enough time to get you out of danger, like running from a scary animal!

Unfortunately, what's happening in today's world is we are living under more prolonged or sustained stress, called **chronic stress**. Chronic stress arises when the triggers of stress do not require instant action. These are events like feeling threatened, big life-changing events such as a pandemic, financial stress, relationship tensions, even feeling unappreciated or unworthy. These sustained events can last for days, months or even years!

What you feel with chronic stress is a constantly present grinding in your mind. You may also feel it churning your stomach, never being quite able to switch off the sense of anxiety (or even dread), but not sure why!

All this grinding and churning affects your day-to-day energy levels, your sleep patterns, maybe your libido[40]! Even everyday functions like digestion can be affected. When you're agonising over a tense conversation or financial issue while sitting down to eat, you're not able to properly digest

---

40 Good article on Medical News Today looks at the effects of stress on the brain, including the effects listed here. It specifically looks at the effects of stress on memory and outlines effects similar to what is experienced during brain fog. Article link — www.medicalnewstoday.com/articles/323445

your food. Specific to long-term fatigue, stress and anxiety are also top of the list of emotional triggers for PEM, as outlined in Chapter 3.

Maybe even more importantly for your fatigue levels and your ability to recuperate is the impact on your immune function. Emotions like stress and anger can negatively affect your immune system. One study found that a burst of anger just five minutes long can cost you five hours of decreased immune function[41]. What could this sustained stress be doing to your immune system at a time when you need it most?

You can start to see the high price paid for every fight, flight or freeze stress response. Even worse is living a lifestyle with frequent intermittent stressors throughout your day. You run the risk of constant activation, flooding your body with stress hormones that provide an instant energy jolt. You might feel hyped and jittery for a while, but then run critically low on energy as it leaves your system. This is the point where you might be tempted to emotionally eat, reaching for those starchy comfort foods for a quick pick-me-up. All this ends in one place…even more fatigue.

Identifying and dealing with your stress

Finding and eliminating unwanted stress in your life is yet another priority, but this is a big one in terms of triggering fatigue.

There are many different forms of stress, including…

1. **Physical stress** — Physical demands on the body, such as PEM-inducing activities, illness and injuries
2. **Psychological stress** — Emotional or mental factors, conditions like anxiety and depression

---

41 This is often quoted as a fact and arises from a 1995 study which looked at the physiological and psychological effects of compassion and anger.

3. **Environmental stress** — External factors including noise, mould, pollution, weather
4. **Social stress** — Lack of connection, conflict within interpersonal relationships

Any of these stress factors has the capability of adding to your fatigue levels. You most likely have a mix of stressors in your life.

What are the top causes of stress in your life right now?

Once you develop awareness around your top contributors to stress, you can start to do something about them.

Stress reduction is highly individual, so you need to find what works for you. Activities that previously provided stress reduction, such as exercise or socialising in person, might no longer be available to you. In this case, your focus needs to shift to ways of relieving stress in a format that works for your current lifestyle. This may involve doing similar activities, but modifying the way you do them to minimise the energy they require.

Here are some ideas for modifications and common stress-busting activities across all four categories.

Physical stress

- Working with your doctor to ease pain and any other underlying physiological stressors, such as existing medical conditions, chronic infections etc.
- Staying hydrated — at least 2 to 3 litres of water a day.
- Knowing your limits and pacing.
- Swapping your normal exercise for gentler versions — e.g. walking not running, yoga or stretching not hitting the gym.

- Exploring gentle, energy building exercises, such as yin yoga, tai chi and qi gong.
- Getting rest, rest and more rest!

Psychological stress

- Spending time in nature, walking on the ground with your bare feet, feeling surrounded by nature.
- Bringing the outside in with house plants or fresh flowers if you are not able to get outside.
- Managing your workload and breaking tasks into achievable chunks — even 15 minutes spent on a task equals progress.
- Swapping any tendencies to keep busy and pack your diary with events with creating more space to calm and slow your mind.
- Practicing meditation, mindfulness and breathing techniques that require little effort.
- Doing the brain dump exercise from the sleep section for that worrying, busy mind.
- Finding professional support — either paid for accessing free services available in your country.
- Cultivating your healing mindset — utilising concepts such as positive focus, gratitude and reframing. (Chapter 8 provides a framework for developing your healing mindset).

Environmental stress

- Removing toxins from your house, such as buying natural cleaning products.

- Stopping the use of strong-smelling and synthetic products, such as air fresheners, perfumes or candles.
- Improving ventilation by opening windows or using a fan.
- Ensuring your home environment is not contaminated with mould. A building biologist or accredited mould remediator can investigate.
- Using a quality water filter to remove contaminants from your drinking water.
- Incorporating houseplants to help improve your air quality (and general good vibes!).

Social stress

- Connecting through a weekly phone call (or video call) with a friend rather than physically meeting. You can set a limit of 10-20 minutes on the days you are feeling fatigue.
- Joining online forums related to fatigue or your condition to find support and understanding.
- Limiting time spent within stressful relationships, setting boundaries, and saying 'no' where necessary. (Chapter 17 provides more help with this point).
- Speaking to a professional therapist to help develop tools and strategies.

Dealing with stress sustainably

Stressed about being stressed? Yes, that's a vicious circle! Rather than exhausting yourself trying to eliminate all sources of stress in your life, a good first step would be to identify the one or two sources that cause the most friction and implement one of the remediations. Over time, you can move on to the next source and so on.

Small reductions in daily stress can lead to massive stress reduction over time. Chief among these priorities is developing your healing mindset, which promotes healing, growth and wellbeing (discussed at length in Chapter 8). Your healing mindset is a natural stress-reliever, creating less tension and more acceptance in your mind. This will have a flow-on effect to the way you view other sources of stress in your life.

4. **Dealing with POTS**

POTS was introduced in Chapter 2 as a condition that is a form of dysautonomia, a disorder of the autonomic nervous system. It commonly accompanies fatigue.

POTS can be a serious condition with symptoms such as:

- Dizziness, light-headedness or vertigo
- Shaking and sweating
- Weakness and fatigue
- Shortness of breath
- Chest pain
- Fainting
- Vomiting
- Heart palpitations
- Headaches
- Poor sleep

It can take a while to find the correct medical diagnosis and an appropriate treatment plan that will help you manage these often-debilitating symptoms.

Smart, wearable technology such as a smart watch or Fitbit can be useful for gathering the data needed to diagnose this condition, such as resting heart rate and heart rate changes when standing and moving.

Once you have a diagnosis, you will work with your medical team to find what works for you. Here is a summary of simple lifestyle changes and formal treatments that others have reported being prescribed by their medical practitioner and having helped with POTS symptoms.

1. **Keeping hydrated** — Drink water in the morning just as you're getting out of bed. Drink the recommended amount during the day (2 to 3 litres per day).
2. **Salt/electrolytes** — Use electrolytes in the morning. Eat salted foods or add extra salt when cooking. Mineral supplementation as prescribed by a health professional.
3. **Compression garments** — Garments such as tights and socks.
4. **Dietary changes** — Keep to a low inflammation diet (e.g. no sugar, flour, dairy or gluten). Eat smaller more frequent meals and regular snacks rather than big meals.
5. **Avoiding triggers such as heat and standing up quickly or for too long** — If heat is a trigger, have cooler showers and sit down in the shower. Use a stool when doing activities such as cooking. Get up slowly from a reclining position.
6. **Beta blockers** — A trained professional such as a doctor or cardiologist might prescribe something like propranolol.
7. **Heart-brain coherence techniques**[42] — A field that looks to manage stress and deepen the connection to your own body, finding harmony

---

42 Heart-brain coherence techniques are often recommended by various functional and integrative doctors. A good site to find out more about this topic is here — www.heartmath.org/research/

or flow between your heart and your brain, using heart rate variability (HRV) to measure it. Activities like breathing exercises and meditation are often recommended to lessen symptoms.

Finding the best treatments for POTS is often trial and error and should always be done under medical supervision.

What works

- **Prioritising healthy lifestyle choices** — With so little energy resources to 'spend' in your day, consciously choose what you want to prioritise. Having lifestyle fundamentals in place will potentially lead to more energy over time.
- **Finding the practitioners who can help** — Lifestyle choices can be supported by good professional care when you find the team that understands fatigue and can adapt to your unique needs.
- **Small changes that develop into good lifestyle habits** — Bit by bit, making small changes and lifestyle improvements that support your fatigue condition in a way that doesn't expect too much from you. Small changes might be prioritising making healthy meals a few times a week, ensuring a consistent bedtime and a good sleep routine, daily walking in the sunshine — even just a few blocks each day. From small changes, big benefits can grow.
- **Test and challenge** — With no set prescribed way of dealing with long-term fatigue, it comes down to finding out what will work best for you. Continuously testing and challenging your choices will mean you eventually settle on a routine that feels good for you.
- **Join forums and ask others what helps** — There are more and more online forums popping up where people dealing with long-term fatigue can collaborate, particularly for the long-COVID community. Joining

these forums will help you find out what other lifestyle choices people are making and can provide ideas and advice for your own situation.

What doesn't work

- **Creating more mental and emotional load**[43] — Guilt and judgements you feel when you don't stick to good lifestyle choices will only add to your fatigue. Instead, try to forgive any transgressions and start again the next day with a clean slate.

- **Relying on one source of lifestyle advice** — Relying on one source, even if they seem to have all the answers, will potentially result in missed opportunities. Long-term fatigue is a complex condition. You will likely need a range of advice. You might use your primary care doctor as a central support, but seek advice from your full range of options, such as professionals, online forums, books and fatigue-related organisations.

- **Trying to change too much too quickly** — Modifying your lifestyle choices is best done over time. Changing too much too quickly can shock your body, make it difficult to ascertain what works and what doesn't, and can lead to difficulty sustaining the change.

---

43 Find self-compassion exercises and free meditation resources here —self-compassion.org/category/exercises/

Chapter 15

Becoming a Pacing Expert

"I was a firefighter in Dunedin, New Zealand for four years before I was hit out of the blue with a diagnosis of chronic fatigue syndrome. Fatigue and brain fog started interfering with my ability to do my job. It's crucially important that I am always fully functioning as we are frequently in life-and-death situations.

At the start, my leader was unsympathetic and even suggested that I wasn't trying hard enough to manage my condition. Luckily, he moved on and the next chief has been a champion. He's provided me with the flexibility I need, and I now work part-time in the mornings, as this is when I'm at my best. I've learnt to pace myself and keep a lower profile on my days off, which means mainly resting. I resented having to do this at the beginning, but have learnt to just embrace this as my new way of life…for now anyway!"

— Keenan, 28, New Zealand

As per the fuller exploration in Chapter 5, pacing is the number one skill that anyone with long-term fatigue will master during their marathon journey. At its heart, pacing is about establishing a routine of activity that works within your current energy levels.

A big component of pacing is understanding your energy envelope, or the amount of energy you have available each day. The first step involves listening to your body to establish your limits, knowing that these can change from day to day. Ideally, you'll get to know these limits well and adapt your lifestyle to your current abilities. If you experience PEM, you will already know well the feedback you receive when you've overdone things, facing the consequences over the days to come. This includes any number of symptoms, including our trusty exhaustion and brain fog!

Becoming a pacing expert is about embracing this strategy for managing your lifestyle and fatigue. It's about understanding your own rules around finite energy and being able to ration your energy to focus on what's most important to you. A large component of this is about understanding how much energy you have available right now, your energy envelope and your physical, mental and emotional triggers for PEM. A full outline of these triggers is available in Chapter 3.

One of the biggest challenges within long-term fatigue is that your energy levels might fluctuate, waxing and waning throughout your days. Earlier chapters asked you to consider your body as a battery and your energy as the charge. With long-term fatigue, your battery is faulty and will need more frequent recharging throughout the day to be able to keep going. Pacing is about listening to your body, identifying your limits and putting in place what's needed to recharge your faulty battery regularly.

It is also about constantly adjusting the amount of activity you take on to accommodate these fluctuations and minimise PEM, even making weekly changes if need be. Unfortunately, adjustments each week are sometimes not practical when you factor in work and other commitments. Frequently, those of us with long-term fatigue find ourselves exhausted trying to keep up with commitments until eventually something must give — hopefully not our sanity!

Pacing is never an exact science and becoming an expert usually involves the odd lapse into fatigue. What you can aim for is a good understanding of where your limits lie and a schedule that accommodates these limits as best you can.

I've developed a process for how you might establish a routine of activity, understanding your limits and scheduling your week. As an expert in pacing, eventually it will become instinctive to balance activity against your current energy levels, learning to say no with more ease when you know it won't serve you well.

There's a lot to consider, so I've broken it down into five steps to make it easier to navigate as suits you.

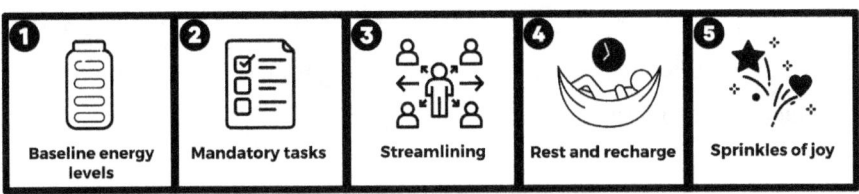

Figure 23 — Five Steps to Balancing Activity and Energy

Step 1 — Baseline energy levels

The first step for managing your week is to get a feel for your baseline level of energy. This is how much energy you have available for activity — most likely a mix of tasks like self-care, working, household chores, responsibilities relating to looking after children, walking your dog, special projects… even social occasions need to be factored in.

You can start by identifying where you place yourself on the energy continuum, assigning a number out of a possible 10. Keep in mind this evaluation is based on your current energy levels, your new normal. Unfortunately, it is not based on the energy you used to have before long-term fatigue, or indeed want to have!

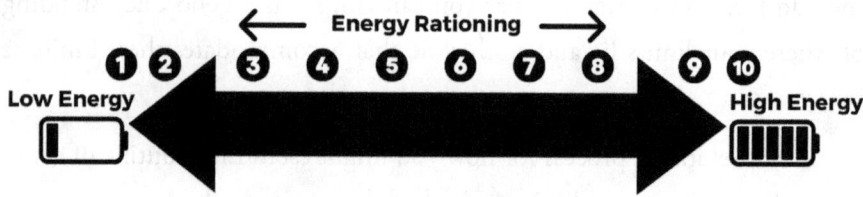

Figure 24 — Energy Continuum

I first introduced this model in Chapter 4, and here is a reminder of each of the points and what they represent.

Low energy (1 or 2 out of 10) — The amount of energy you have when your battery is low. You might be virtually bed-bound with small amounts of movement tolerated. Use of a wheelchair might be required. Simple activities such as getting up and showering require rest afterward.

Energy rationing (anywhere between 3 to 8 out of 10) — In between low and high energy, you have a certain amount of energy to use in the day. You might have less energy than is required to work full-time, but enough to do common household tasks, taking short walks outside, etc. Completing activities often requires rest afterwards and too much exertion results in PEM.

High energy (9 or 10 out of 10) — The amount of energy you have when your battery is at full charge. 'Normal' activities are possible, such as work, social occasions and exercise and you do not get PEM after completing these activities.

Considering an average week, what number would you assign yourself out of 10 for your current energy levels?

Your baseline energy out of 10 will reveal where you are on your energy continuum and provide guidance as to what activities are available to you.

As a general guide:

If you are low energy (1 or 2) — You are heavily fatigued and most likely do not have the energy for anything but the basics of self-care.

If you are towards the low end of energy rationing (3, 4 or 5) — You can plan activities, but might not have confidence you will be able to fulfil them. It is vitally important to listen to your body's limits in this stage. Prioritise getting adequate rest and recharge between activities.

If you are towards the high end of energy rationing (6, 7 or 8) — You can plan activities with more confidence, knowing that there is good chance you will be able to complete them. This is a danger zone and where many people overdo it, only to fall back into PEM or a longer-term crash. In this stage, you can enjoy your energy, but your rest and recharge routine is still your priority.

If you are high energy (9 or 10) — You're close to your full energy allocation and can plan activities with confidence. You can use this time to push yourself more than you normally would and even incorporate more activities that fill your cup. Examples of this include scheduling social occasions, taking on a special project, doing more physically challenging activities, or even enjoying some new learning.

This is a rough guide, and you'll instinctively get to know your own body and limits as time goes by.

When you have high baseline energy (anything 7 or above), this can be another danger zone as you rush to do all the wonderful things that have recently been unavailable to you. Too often you might find yourself overdoing it, back into that crash and burn cycle, which can feel devastating after a taste of freedom.

Operating with caution is always the best strategy when you're in a high-energy state, especially at the beginning when you are getting used to your limits.

From this place of caution, the next step is around working out what activities absolutely must be incorporated into your schedule.

Step 2 — Mandatory tasks

Once you have a baseline understanding of your current energy levels, pacing involves identifying what absolutely **must be done.**

This may involve:

- Self-care such as showering, grooming, getting dressed
- Work requirements
- Appointments such as doctors' visits
- Responsibilities like picking your children up from school
- Caring arrangements such as childcare, parental care and pet care
- Practical tasks like grocery shopping, cooking, washing and cleaning
- School work, homework, other types of learning

What's on your mandatory task list? Make your list now!

Step 3 — Streamlining

The previous step identified all the things that absolutely must be in your schedule. Now you can look at what is going to **help you get these tasks done**.

Examples include:

- **Finding efficiencies** — Finding ways to save energy and become more efficient.
  Examples include: using technology to work from home rather than travelling, saving commute time and energy; attending appointments over the phone or via telehealth rather than in person; batch-cooking for the week rather than making individual meals.

- **Delegating/outsourcing** — Getting tasks done through other people.
  Examples include: asking someone else to clean or do your groceries, grocery shopping online and getting them delivered or buying pre-cooked meals; asking someone to do research for you and give you the summary only; lightening your load at work by allowing others to do non-essential tasks; sharing pick-up and driving responsibilities with another parent.

- **Letting things go** — Focusing on what's important and allowing the rest to not matter as much.
  Examples include: accepting your house may be untidy for a while when you have extremely low energy; identifying any perfectionist tendencies and allowing them to ease; divesting in social occasions that don't serve you.

This is an important step to make sure you are conserving your energy, using it for the things that matter most. This can help you avoid wasting energy on tasks that are not so important or that can wait until you have more energy available.

Once you have this in order, you can fill your calendar with what you absolutely **must do** first.

Where can you streamline your task list and make life just that little bit easier? Go through your mandatory task list and make some suggestions.

Step 4 — Rest and recharge

Next, look at what will assist you to get through the week and achieve your mandatory tasks — your rest and recharge routine.

Rest and recharge can be many things:

- Sleep
- Listening to music or podcasts
- Watching TV
- Time with a certain person or pets
- Practicing self-care activities, such as meditation or stretching
- Gentle exercise to promote relaxation
- Time in a dark room with no mental stimulation (sensory deprivation)

Over time, you will get to know your limits and when your battery needs a charge. Your rest breaks are precious. Therefore, it is crucial that you protect this time throughout each and every day. This only becomes reality when you factor this time into your schedule.

Rest and recharge can prevent further fatigue and provide the boost of energy needed to do the activities that mean the most to you. If they are not scheduled, they can tend to fall to the wayside, leaving you vulnerable to a crash.

Ideally, you'll be able to schedule these breaks *before* you start to feel fatigued to give yourself the best chance of not experiencing PEM. If you are still adjusting to your limits, when you start feeling fatigued, then take this as your cue to take a break. This is all good feedback that allows you to adjust your pace and conserve your precious energy throughout the day.

What gives you the rest and recharge you need? How do you need to schedule this throughout your day?

Step 5 — Sprinkles of joy

You've now identified all the things you absolutely must do and found ways to make them easier to achieve. You've also scheduled your battery's rest and recharge time.

The last piece of the scheduling puzzle involves planning what brings a smile to your face — your sprinkles of joy! The science behind happiness and joy is clear — it is a mandatory part of any healthy lifestyle. Feeling joy regularly has many benefits that you need for managing long-term fatigue, such as boosting your mood, strengthening your immune system, helping fight stress and pain, not to mention helping with all the emotional difficulties that frequently accompany long-term chronic conditions[44].

It doesn't have to be much. It might be:

...a phone call with a loved one.

---

44 An interesting healthline article outlines how happiness and joy affects your brain and body, including all the benefits that assist people with long-term chronic conditions. Article link —www.healthline.com/health/affects-of-joy

…social time with family and friends.

…cuddle time with someone special, your pet or even a stuffed toy will do!

…a delicious meal you're looking forward to.

…listening to uplifting music or a podcast.

…a beautiful scent, such as lighting a candle or the abundant smells in nature.

…sitting in the morning sun for 10 minutes a day for a boost of vitamin D.

Anything that brings you joy is okay! It's all about finding those little moments that make you feel connected and alive.

You might find it easy to forget about joy when caught up with the intricacies of pacing and fatigue. It's a condition with many challenges and limitations, but that's not all life is about. Finding your sprinkles of joy will most likely become the highlights of your week.

Over time, your brain will become wired to automatically seek out your sprinkles, perhaps without you even being aware!

Where are your sprinkles of joy? Place them regularly throughout your week.

A skillset for life

This is my five-step process for building your weekly schedule that incorporates all the important elements of pacing.

Eventually you will instinctively and automatically balance your activity against your current energy levels. You won't always be perfect. You may even overdo it on occasion. Becoming an expert in pacing is about incrementally learning your limits for the long-term. If you follow these steps for a whole month, I'll be ready to graduate you!

Dealing with fatigue can seem like you are forced to become a pacing expert, but a better way to look at that you are developing a skillset that will serve you well for the rest of your life. Indeed, it is often pointed out to me that you don't need to be fatigued to benefit — this is a magnificent skillset that everyone can adopt in order to build more sustainability into their life.

What works

- **Prioritising until it becomes natural** — Like any skill, it can take time to learn how to prioritise your day. The key to this skill is learning what priorities need to be done, doing them and then being happy with what you have been able to do.

- **Assessing your daily energy and working to that limit** — Having your schedule done and visible so you can move towards a routine is one thing. But you also need to listen to your body and work to your daily limits. Where possible, have backup plans in place for the days when your energy fluctuates and you have less energy than usual. Your aim is to find a routine of activity that allows you to break out of any boom-and-bust cycles you have entered and minimise the occurrence of PEM.

- **Breaking tasks into smaller, more manageable chunks** — Rather than trying to do the full task all at once, it's often better to do a short amount. This might mean doing 15 minutes of activity and then resting. If you repeat this four times over your day, you have an hour of activity. This is a better result than sitting for an hour with a task that results in PEM afterwards.

- **Resting regularly** — This is about knowing how best to rest and recharge, and doing it as often as required throughout your day. On your worst days, it may be you can't do anything visual such as watching TV or reading, so listening to a podcast or music with your eyes closed becomes your alternative. Over time you will learn to work with what your body needs in the moment to get adequate rest.

What doesn't work

- **Pushing yourself** — Except on the odd occasion when it's important and you absolutely must, pushing yourself should be avoided. It will most likely result in PEM and an even harder time the next day.

- **Ignoring your new limits** — Long-term fatigue comes with new limits, your new normal, compared to your previous activity levels. Unfortunately, this is the reality and ignoring it is never a good strategy. When scheduling, it's better to under-commit and be able to do more than expected than over-commit and feel bad or like you're letting yourself and others down.

- **Engaging in unhelpful thinking** — You might schedule your week, but at times experience lower energy or PEM. You might then not be able to follow through completely. Your pattern may be to beat yourself up about this mentally and engage the range of unhelpful thought patterns outlined in Chapter 7. Unfortunately, some days these energy fluctuations will be out of your control. A longer-term goal is to accept this as a fact, and implement acceptance and self-compassion rather than judgement.

Chapter 16
Moving with Care, Not Out of Obligation

"I've been an active gym-goer for most of my adult life, but after long-COVID my energy levels no longer allow exercise and I've dropped my gym membership. Instead, I've found an online yoga class with a trainer called Suzy Bolt who has a tailored class specifically for long-COVID, including rest and meditation in between poses.

After starting with Suzy, I felt better immediately — physically but also fewer mental judgements. I now do three yoga sessions a week along with a gentle walk each morning and 10 minutes of meditation before bedtime. It's been a sanity-saver."

— Jose, 42, Brazil

Most of us discover intense physical activity and long-term fatigue do not mix. Exercise becomes a conundrum. On one hand, it is good to move your body, and your fatigue can feel even worse if you don't. On the other hand, exercise is often not tolerated and not recommended when it induces PEM. A conundrum indeed!

Current research just keeps on revealing the devastating effects of physical activity and Graded Exercise Therapy (GET) when PEM is present[45]. PEM — that cycle of overdoing it one day, crashing and burning the next — can become distressing at the extremes. Constantly triggering PEM can also make your symptoms exponentially worse. No matter how fit or active you were previously, your body can have an adverse reaction to even the slightest amount of physical exertion. This can lead to disastrous consequences for your future self.

PEM can feel like you are walking an invisible line. There is a magic, unknown amount of activity that you can do in a day and not face repercussions for days later. But the rules can also seem to change daily. You often won't know this amount of activity that can be tolerated until you cross that invisible line and are left paying the price.

Managing your expectations around what you can and cannot do is one of the most difficult aspects of dealing with long-term fatigue. For a lot of us, we were once very active and expect a lot from our bodies. You might find your mindset is fixed on how much you 'should' be able to do. You can feel let down by your body and frustrated at your current situation. Your own body can even become your enemy! Carrying these feelings can be exhausting.

Mourning your body's previous capabilities is understandable. There is a grief around letting go that reaches beyond the activity you can't do right now. It can cut deep to the heart of who you are, your very being, particularly if you are an active person.

---

45 Emerge Australia is a good resource for keeping up with the latest research around ME/CFS and long-COVID. Their regular newsletter provides links to research articles and other helpful resources. Find out more at: emerge.org.au

Yet holding on to this previous identity does not help your healing. What *does* help healing is letting go of what you once were able to do and accepting your current reality. This doesn't have to be a permanent acceptance, just an acknowledgment of your current physical limitations and what's within your capability right now.

It can take time to develop this acceptance and it may be a new way of thinking for you. Overall, you are looking for an easier way — a more healing mindset that will support your current capability for movement.

'Moving with care, not out of obligation' is a mindset that promotes healing, not stress. It's about establishing what you *can* do, rather than mourning what you *can't*. It's also about keeping your body as active as possible, within the limits currently available to you. It's even about turning any anger you have at your body into support and gratitude for getting you through until now.

Careful movement involves gentler activities that provide mental and physical benefit, but where you have minimal chance of paying for your effort in the days that follow. You can try the following as a start:

- **Stretching and practicing forms of gentle yoga (seated/reclining poses).** These are great for encouraging deep diaphragmatic breathing, which is both soothing and relaxing. They are also effective at managing stress levels.
- **Walking, particularly on flat surfaces.** Walking outside helps you feel part of the world and at one with nature. It provides a hit of vitamin D (particularly in the morning), which is crucial for good health. It's also great for managing stress levels.

It might 'cost' some of your energy, but these gentle forms of exercise have many benefits. They help maintain your muscle mass and strength, as well as your overall health. Moving also releases endorphins, helping your mood, stress levels and quality of sleep.

Every person is different, and each day may have different rules. Moving with care and finding the activity that is right for your body can be trial and error at the beginning.

When you are ready to begin, try starting with something achievable, such as five minutes of walking per day on a flat surface. You can then slowly — *slowly* — increase the pace and duration over time if that feels available to you. If five minutes is too much to start with, try one minute. If you're confined to bed or a wheelchair, then maybe just some basic arm or leg lifts are your movement for the day. Again, I emphasise to always go slowly. The idea is to *enjoy* the feeling of movement and be content with whatever you are able to achieve.

I always advocate discussing any changes with your primary care doctor. More enlightened practitioners recognise that even moderate exercise is not supported with your current fatigue levels and the associated PEM after-shocks. They will advise prioritising mobility as much as possible, but not to the point that it triggers distress. Towards the end of your marathon journey when you have reached a level of recovery that no longer includes PEM, they may refer you to a qualified exercise physiologist to craft a useful regime that works within your limits. Before then, the invisible PEM line and moving targets make for a difficult equation to manage, one where only you can judge what you will and will not tolerate.

Sometimes practitioners in our cracked medical systems give bad advice! Be alert if you are being pushed towards physical activity, particularly GET, which is still recommended by some practitioners. GET helps with the deconditioning that occurs following inactivity, bedrest or a sedentary lifestyle, but as mentioned before and worth stating again, PEM is **not** deconditioning and should not be treated as such.

Never allow anyone to make you feel like you should be doing more than you are physically capable. As exhausting as it might sound, it is in your own best interest to push back on recommendations around too much or too intense activity (especially GET) in the earlier stages of your fatigue. Not all practitioners are aware that exercise can be harmful to those of us experiencing PEM. Until standardised fatigue treatment advice trickles down in a more systemic fashion, it can be hit or miss as to what is recommended. I urge you to trust in your own intuition and seek out those gems, the more enlightened practitioners.

Gradually over time, you can expect more activity to be available to you. As you navigate the marathon of improvement, the benefits of careful movement become exponential. You will learn your limits, leading to fewer crashes and PEM side effects.

Your goal is simply to keep as active as tolerated. And while this is the best you can do right now, your healing mindset knows it won't always be this way.

What works

- **Gentle exercise done with care** — Look for activities that provide mental and physical benefit but have minimal impact on your energy levels in the days that follow. These could be:
    - Stretching
    - Gentle yoga, particularly seated and reclining poses
    - Walking, particularly on flat surfaces
    - Tai chi with slow fluid movements

- **Letting go of your old fitness expectations** — It doesn't matter if you once ran marathons, or you used to be a super-hero full of energy. This is about working within your current reality. This will free up your headspace to stop the exhausting judgements and focus on what really matters: getting the most out of your days. You can start slow, even just five minutes a day, and work up to what is sustainable for your body.

- **Finding the joy in movement** — The movement in your day, such as daily walks in the fresh air, can be the activity you look forward to most. It becomes a joy when you know it's within your limits. It also provides benefits such as stress relief, increased mobility and social connection.

What doesn't work

- **Moving out of obligation** — Stop yourself from pushing or listening to the echoes of what you used to, or 'should' be able to do. This leads to an exhausting mindset and will most likely result in PEM, both of which are detrimental to your current situation.

- **Making rigid plans** — You will have good days and bad days. Making plans to exercise, by yourself or with someone else, then not being able to keep those plans can be upsetting. Instead, you can communicate your desire to exercise, but leave the door open to assess your energy level on the day.

- **Allowing a practitioner to 'prescribe' exercise before your body is ready** — As referenced in Chapter 11, the medical community hasn't yet caught up with an understanding of PEM, nor provided a recommended approach to exercise with long-term fatigue. Be careful of recommendations to work with therapists and GET when you are still experiencing PEM. You will need to decide for yourself how much and what type of exercise your condition can tolerate.

Chapter 17
Building Your Supportive Team

"I've needed to shelve my social butterfly tendencies for a while as I rest and heal. I used to love going out for dinner, but now one of my good friends comes to me. We usually just order in and watch a funny movie. I'm so grateful for the loyalty of this friend who never judges my house being a mess, or the fact I haven't even brushed my hair today!

If you can find someone to be there for you in this way, then treasure that friendship. In some ways, my condition has made our bond even stronger, and I know how lucky I am to have this unconditional support."

— Maya, 36, Australia

Let's talk about how to build your supportive team. It's a team effort to get you back to full health and the most resilient among us tend to have a good understanding of when we need support and who we can best get it from.

We ended Chapter 10 (managing the people in your life) by identifying a goal. Long term, your goal is for your team to support you as you get back on your feet and find your health again. Short term, you are looking to enjoy your life to the best of your ability.

As we know, living with long-term fatigue can change the rules. Where you could once be a valuable contributor, you now might need to ask for help. If you are a giving type of person and not used to receiving, it can be confronting to have to ask for support, but you might be surprised at how happy people are that they can do something for you. If people don't want to, or can't help you, then maybe they are not right to be on your team.

Your team will also be made up of paid professionals. Building the team of practitioners to support you is just as important as trying to bring your friends into the fold. If your friends and family can't meet some of your needs, you might be open to paying someone to help. If that's not affordable, you can investigate other methods of getting the support you need, such as online support groups or local meetups.

The goal becomes building the team of people around you that provide you with what you need right now. This often involves learning to advocate for yourself. Many people, including friends, family, workmates and even the medical community, will not understand your condition. This requires education, conversations that can feel exhausting and that may or may not draw out understanding and support.

This is where advocating for yourself is also about setting healthy boundaries with the people around you. Over time you can develop the skill and strength to unapologetically say '*no*' to what drains your energy as a non-negotiable. This opens the door to saying '*yes*' to what *will* support you in building up your energy again.

Let's talk about what you can do to meet this goal and build your supportive team, including my three-step process to start you off.

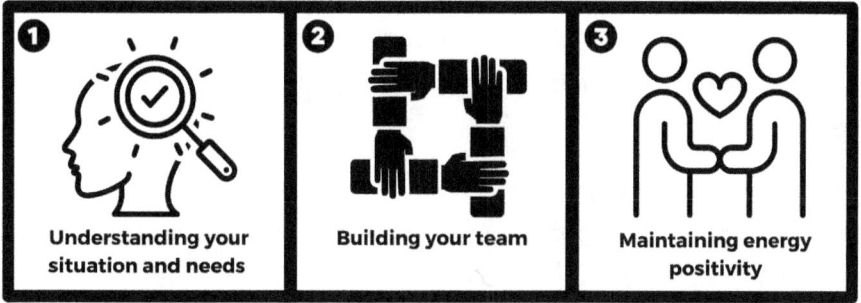

Figure 25 — 3 Steps to Building Your Supportive Team

Step 1 — Understanding your own situation and needs from others

The first step to building your team and drawing those healthy boundaries is clarifying your rules of engagement — how you actually want to interact with others.

Often this involves overcoming those energy-depleting habituated behaviours that might be ingrained. Examples of these include:

- Saying yes when you really want to say no.
- Bottling up resentments and other negative emotions (until they come to a tipping point and burst out)
- Spiralling conversations that focus on venting and negativity
- Taking on the negative emotions of others and feeling drained as a result
- Tolerating certain situations because you don't want to face confrontation or don't have a model for how you would prefer it to be instead

You no longer have the energy for these behaviours! It is time for a change.

This step is about getting clear on what you need from your team and feeling the confidence to ask for it. This starts with your own self-understanding. I do recognise that it can be difficult to understand exactly what is going on for yourself when you have a condition such as fatigue, much less feel able to articulate it to other people. To the best of your ability, you need to try.

It starts with asking yourself what you need from others. At my peak fatigue, for example, I needed support, people to listen and understand, and at times just to be left alone!

In figuring out what you might need, consider if you need:

- To talk it out with another person
- To have someone (or something) just listen
- To feel more connection with others
- To share in the experience of others also dealing with long-term conditions
- To write it down and get it out of your head
- To find professional advice and support

The decision may not be immediately obvious, so four general tips for getting clearer on your needs include:

1. Writing down your thoughts and feelings in a document or a journal
2. Speaking to a professional such as a counsellor or psychologist
3. Engaging in online forums with other people going through a similar experience to find out what support they access
4. Reading books like this to spark ideas!

Being clearer on your own needs means you can become more transparent in the way you communicate to those around you, confidently saying what you need to say. It will stop the energy-depleting behaviours you may have fallen into in the past, such as the automatic yes or bottling up your emotions. Instead, it provides a set of criteria to evaluate what you need and who can provide this to you.

What are your needs? Outline what you currently need from others.

Step 2 — Building your team

Once you have a clearer idea of your needs, the next step is to build that supportive team around you.

This is always going to be a mix of people:

1. Trusted friends and family who can be relied upon
2. People who have experienced your condition and can relate
3. Paid professionals who can give you solid advice and guidance with no agenda of their own
4. Groups of people totally unrelated who don't ask too much of you but help with a sense of connection

Think about who you need on your team. It can be family, your mum and dad, siblings, cousins, your partner, a pet, close friends, your doctor or psychologist, a friend from a club or interest group.

Even keeping a diary of your own thoughts can provide you with a feeling of support.

Your supportive team can come from anywhere. My dog was a constant support on the days I just couldn't get out of bed!

Who do you need on your team? Create your list now!

Step 3 — Maintaining energy positivity

Once you have your team in place, it becomes about finding ways of utilising them to meet your needs, balancing out what feels draining versus what lifts you up. This is about having those healthy boundaries in place so you can focus on letting go of the energy-depleting behaviours and conserving your energy for where it's most needed.

Communication is key at this stage. Setting healthy boundaries means being ready and clear with those messages from Step 1 around what you need right now.

Here are three tips around healthy boundary-setting and maintaining energy positivity:

1. **Productive conversations** — Conversations with a good friend or family member where you're both used to being able to vent may suddenly drain and exhaust you. When you need a change of rules, turn to productive conversations (outlined in Chapter 8).

    Rather than sitting in negativity or pure venting, such productive conversations deepen your understanding and assist you to reframe your experiences in a more positive light. It might be you need to teach your team (including yourself!) how to have these ongoing productive conversations.

2. **Saying no** — Instead of the automatic yes, you can find respectful and appropriate ways of giving yourself space and saying no. This involves

getting used to making statements like, *"Thank you and I'll get back to you on that"* or *"I can't make that, but hope you have a great time"*. Another great statement is, *"For my sanity, I'm implementing a 24-hour decision-making window!"*[46]

3. **Pick your timing** — Conversations need to occur when you are best able to have them. It's counterproductive to initiate conversations when you're fatigued, emotional or experiencing brain fog, for example. In this state, there is a fine line between getting the support you need and alienating those around you!

It's much more productive to wait until you have the most clarity in your thinking along with the emotional energy to take this on. I've found it useful to flag that I'm not available for a particular conversation right now but would like to pick it up again when I'm rested. While this might seem jarring at first, those close to you will become used to this rhythm over time.

What you can control is being as open, honest and clear as possible. Creating this space and putting in boundaries is a way of interacting with greater integrity with those around you. It lessens the amount of resentment you may feel towards others when you don't feel like you're getting your needs met. And remember, this is all about keeping your team energy positive rather than an energy drain!

How can you maintain energy positivity in your life? Outline one or two strategies that will make the most difference.

---

[46] A great resource for boundary-setting is the book *Boundary Boss* by Terri Cole. Much of my boundary-setting advice is sourced originally from Terri's work.

Skills for life

Healthy boundary-setting and maintaining energy positivity in your relationships is not just for when you're fatigued. This is a skill for all of us all the time!

Productive conversations can be a life-changing concept, akin to adopting a growth rather than fixed mindset[47]. These conversations can be with either another person or with yourself. Keeping a journal or diary (or any type of writing) can help structure your thoughts. I've always found once something is written down and out of my head, this provides clarity and prevents me from ruminating over and over on the same topic.

> Keep in mind all of this is a conversation, or even a series of conversations, where both parties are seeking to feel seen, heard and understood. If you are struggling with how to communicate your experience, don't forget your bonus resource, which provides the scripts and conversation starters you need to begin having these important conversations.
>
> You can get your copy at: www.sarahvizer.com/tootiredtothink

What works

- **Communicating your current situation to those close to you** — It can be difficult putting into words what is going on with you, but being able to do this gives the people around you a chance to understand. Some will step up and some won't be able to, but you first have to give them the opportunity to support you.

---

[47] The work by Carol Dweck in her book 'Mindset' is an incredible exploration of what a growth mindset entails.

- **Seeking positive impact** — This is about identifying the few people who have the most positive impact on your life and using your energy resources wisely to invest in these relationships.

- **Letting go of relationships that drain your energy** — Some people build you up and some drain you. It's not always easy, but limiting time with the drainers and focusing on energy positive people frees up your precious energy.

- **Adding professional support to your team** — If possible, bringing in professionals who can support your physical and emotional needs will help ensure you are getting the right treatment at this time. It can also be easier to deal with a professional who doesn't have any agendas of their own, rather is there to help you in their own specific capacity.

What doesn't work

- **Allowing others to drain your energy** — Taking control over who you have around you is a proactive way of conserving the precious energy that you do have. Where you don't have a choice, find methods of shielding your energy through means such as setting boundaries, having productive conversations or even just switching off.

- **Being closed off to receiving help** — It can be difficult to ask for help even when you most need it, but not asking prevents others from supporting you in ways they may want to. Keeping yourself open to help when it is offered (or even being brave enough to ask!) delivers much-needed support and allows the other person the joy of being of service.

Chapter 18
Navigating Work Situations

"I'm a single mum who works in customer service. I've been lucky with the flexibility offered in my job as I've been able to spend a year slowly increasing from eight hours a week to my current twenty hours.

I've also had some challenges. I needed to change positions to accommodate my employer's requirements. I also negotiated a hold on my mortgage payments for six months during this transition.

At the beginning, I worked Mondays and Thursdays and found even working eight hours a week a challenge. It required a lot of brain power and resulted in a crash on the days in between shifts, making it difficult to be present with my family. It became a huge learning curve and I learnt to protect those days off — no medical appointments, no housework, just resting and focusing on what brought me peace and joy.

I now work four lots of five-hour shifts over the week and have found a good balance in work and lifestyle. I find I can tolerate the workdays with almost no PEM on days off. It's taken the best part of a year, but I now have energy left over to be with my family and still focus on activities that fill my cup."

— Tina, 38, Australia

What do you do when you're too sick to work, but you need the income to survive? This is the challenging situation so many of us face when dealing with long-term fatigue.

Dealing with fatigue can be extremely difficult in any work environment. It often involves an increase in exhausting medical appointments when you need to provide evidence of your condition. It can involve a burden of proof with insurance companies (if you are lucky enough to have insurance). It can also involve pushing yourself beyond what is achievable and (should be) reasonable for practical reasons such as you need a job and/or emotional reasons such as you don't want to let anyone down.

One of the biggest issues becomes the unknown timeframe of the condition. It is extremely difficult to estimate when long-term fatigue will resolve and therefore when you'll be ready to come back to work.

In my case, with no idea what was in store, I originally took two weeks leave because I was feeling completely burnt out. After two weeks, it became apparent that I was in no fit state to return to work and my leave was extended. This went on for a while, every month extending my leave as the true extent of my fatigue made itself known.

Workplaces can forgive you being sick for a while. They can forgive a less hidden, more visible illness that leaves physical traces such as cancer, a broken bone or any issue requiring surgery. The challenge can be workplaces being patient long-term when the effects of your condition are for the most part hidden, and you don't have clarity on when you'll realistically be able to return to your position. After a year of leave, my workplace made the call to end the uncertainty and terminate my employment. It was a relief as I was barely able to leave my bedroom at that stage, but it also came with its own stages of grief.

My story is not unique. After reviewing my research into stories of others navigating fatigue, a number of patterns emerged for how people negotiate their work situation with a long-term fatigue condition.

For many, their best bet is negotiating with their current employer and seeking flexibility within their current arrangement. They reduce their hours or take a leave of absence from their work, using leave entitlements such as sick and annual leave. They return to work with a phased approach after a period away. Some hold insurance and can prove their condition to receive benefit. Some can lighten their responsibilities, or even embrace the benefits of doing only what's absolutely necessary for a while. Ideally for these situations, you will have the support of your leaders.

For others, the options are not as bright. Some employees are pushed for an early retirement. Those on contracts do not have them renewed and face the daunting task of finding new work while simultaneously dealing with their condition. They may apply for government support and find themselves navigating the various disability systems around the world — or lack thereof. The self-employed face similar options around working with their insurance or taking leave. They may have flexibility to work part-time, or outsource, even stepping away for a period.

For my own situation, I was not able to work for many years and resorted to using my savings — going backwards but feeling privileged I had a buffer to fall back on. I've since started my own business, as this offers more flexibility than working for an employer and allows for my continued fatigue.

Your choices around how to navigate your work situation can be difficult to make. A full summary of options reported by people facing long-term fatigue include:

1. **Negotiating with your current employer**
- Lightening your workload — e.g. seeking greater support from your team, postponing non-urgent projects, requesting flexibility on hours and deadlines.
- Using accrued leave entitlements as and when needed — e.g. sick leave, annual leave.
- Taking a defined leave of absence — e.g. three-month period using any accrued leave entitlements and/or leave without pay.
- Returning to work with a phased approach.
- Making an insurance claim.

2. **Changing arrangements with your current employer**
- Dropping your days and hours worked, such as going part-time.
- Changing roles or taking up job-sharing options.
- Going on lighter duties for a period.
- Working from home for a period.

3. **Leaving your current employer**
- Leaving your current job altogether.
- Applying for government support — e.g. disability payments.
- Options like taking early retirement.
- Finding another job that suits your condition better — e.g. slower paced, more flexibility, part-time options.

- Starting your own business.
- Support provided by family and/or partner.

There is also the option for some with milder forms of fatigue to make no significant changes, rather carrying on the best they can in their current work situation. In this case, it can be helpful to still negotiate as much flexibility as possible within your current arrangement. What you don't want to do is push yourself further than you can tolerate, worsen your fatigue symptoms and potentially extend recovery timelines.

There may be alternate paths available to you, but these are the big-ticket choices others have made. Next, we look at how best to handle your work changes once you establish the choice that is best for you out of the options available.

Navigating work changes

When making any changes to your work situation, whether you work for yourself or for someone else, the first order of business is to document as much of your medical condition as you can manage. As part of this, it is important to have your primary care doctor in place and build your medical team to obtain a clear and documented diagnosis and treatment plan. The benefit of having this team and medical documentation in place is you have 'proof' around your 'fit for work' status, from which you can then apply for leave, insurance and/or government support.

Making changes when you work for someone else usually involves communication with multiple parties. Your primary care doctor is the person to help substantiate any requests for flexibility and sign you off from work, as well as help you transition back into the workplace when you are ready. They can provide you with important documents such as a 'fit for work' note and advise on how many hours you can do within a set timeframe.

If you have access to occupational health in your workplace, they will most likely have a better understanding of the demands of your role and what is realistic. Engaging them can support you to ensure your employer works within your doctor's recommendations.

With your documentation in place, you can then start negotiating with the relevant parties. General advice for negotiating with employers and insurance claims is as follows:

1. Have as much medical documentation as you can to substantiate your condition.
2. Be as clear and honest in your communication as possible. Keep lines of communication open with all parties — including leaders, human resources and occupational health.
3. Be clear on the outcomes you are seeking. Are you looking for lighter duties, a leave of absence, part-time arrangement, gradual return to work?
4. Try to create flexibility in your arrangement and negotiate any accommodations you might need, such as regular working from home days, flexible hours.

Transitioning back to work

Like any changing situation, when you are ready to transition back to work it will take time to settle back in. You will most likely have some extra challenges arising from your condition, such as knowing your energy levels might fluctuate. There will be times you need to rest after a crash.

Start by creating as much of a buffer in the arrangements as you can to accommodate these fluctuations. In your communication, you might be able to stress the need to see how things go at the beginning. Obtaining clear recommendations from your medical team will support this.

A good approach that has worked for others is a phased return. This involves gradually stepping up your days and hours slowly over a set period. The more flexibility you can build into this arrangement the better because you will not know how your body will tolerate the change in the beginning. It's always best to start small and build up gradually, assessing each step as you go. You might even need to pause an increase in steps if you find yourself struggling.

It becomes critical to manage your energy over the week as you establish your routine. A phased return might include shorter hours over more days, at least in the beginning, lessening the risk of a perpetual boom-and-bust cycle.

Depending on your best times to work — mornings, afternoons or evenings — a phased return may start with two hours a day and gradually increase to five (or more). You may start out spreading it over the week, such as Monday, Wednesday, Friday with rest days in between to aid recovery.

You might find you crash on the days in between, especially at the beginning, but long-term the goal is to build a sustainable lifestyle where you enjoy your life, not crash on your days off.

General advice for transitioning back into the workplace after a time away includes…

1. **Scale back your other activity** — Expect work to take over much of your energy when first starting back. You can help this by cutting back on your other commitments and scaling back your personal life at least temporarily while you adjust.
2. **Use your expert pacing skills** — As an expert in pacing, you can now manage your energy levels and be more deliberate when saying yes. You

can also not be afraid to say no while you get used to a new work rhythm and routine.

3. **Prioritise rest and sleep** — At the start, you will most likely experience a lot more sensory overload than you have been used to, which can lead to fatigue, brain fog and PEM. Work out a rhythm that includes as much rest and sleep as you need to manage these effects.

4. **Keep stress in your life as low as possible** — Transitioning back to work will already be providing an increased stress level. Maybe easier said than done, but keeping the rest of your life as low a stress level as possible will lessen the chance of more fatigue and PEM.

5. **Lower your expectations of yourself** — It's okay for things to be less than perfect for a while, especially as you are transitioning. Your healing mindset can forgive a messy house or less participation in family events over this time. Give yourself the time you need to establish your new routine and responsibilities.

6. **Be open in your need for flexibility** — Things may not go as planned and you might not able to increase your hours each week. There might even be periods where you need to pause or step back. Being honest with yourself and understanding your own needs comes first. Then you can keep those lines of communication open with those around you and express your needs more easily.

One final consideration when dealing with long-term fatigue and changes in your work situation involves your financial requirements. In many cases, changes in work circumstances will result in a decrease in your income for a while. This can be a difficult situation to navigate and might involve asking some tough questions. Examples of these include:

1. Realistically, how many hours a day and days a week do I need to work to support my lifestyle?
2. What expenses can I cut down (and not miss) to reduce the amount of money I require (and therefore work I have to do)?
3. If times got tough, what assets could I sell or who could I ask for assistance?

While these may be tough questions at the beginning, after a bit of consideration there may be ways of simplifying life to free up capital and not rely on the income from a previously full-time job. This can go a long way towards providing breathing room as you get your condition in check.

What works

- **Documenting your medical history** — Working with your primary care doctor, keeping records of all aspects of your condition, including your diagnosis (if you have one), and recommended treatment plan.
- **Start small and gradually build up** — General advice when transitioning back into the workforce is to start as small as you can and build up gradually, including phased returns and part-time arrangements.
- **Find a location to rest during the day, if needed** — Scouting a location for downtime ahead of time takes the pressure off when you need some rest. Examples include getting out into nature such as nearby park, using a sick bay to lie down, or finding a spare room or office to sit quietly.

What doesn't work

- **Promising exact timeframes** — Long-term fatigue can be difficult to predict, so building flexibility into your arrangement gives you room to move if needed around timeframes for leave, transition periods etc.

- **Transitioning too quickly** — Starting back with too many hours a day or too many days a week can lead to fatigue, brain fog and PEM. Work with professionals such as your doctor and occupational health support to establish a transition plan that will work within your current situation.

Chapter 19
Ways of Feeling Mindful

"Dealing with effects of fibromyalgia winds me up so tight at times I can barely breathe. I find this condition so frustrating. I'm bursting with rage one minute and in tears the next. I know my body is just not designed for this long-term stress and it's all adding to my fatigue levels.

Lately I've been using an app on my phone called Calm. It guides me and provides regular meditations, which has been exactly what I need. I even fall asleep during some of the meditations and wake up feeling more refreshed than just sleeping. I've had less frustration and tears lately and recommend this app to anyone who needs help rebalancing their emotional state."

— Ute, 25, Germany

Both mindfulness and meditation provide deep relaxation, as well as balance and harmony to your body, mind and spirit. And who wouldn't want some of that!?

There are differences between the two:

- **Mindfulness** is a quality of paying attention in a moment. It involves being able to hover calmly and objectively over your thoughts, feelings and emotions[48].
- **Meditation** is more of a practice where you are looking to connect with, be with and recharge yourself. It uses a combination of mental and physical techniques (such as concentrating on your breathing or repetition of a mantra) for the purpose of reaching a heightened level of spiritual awareness[49].

When dealing with long-term fatigue, you've seen that strong negative emotions are often present. Emotions like frustration and overwhelm are frequently the cause of even more fatigue. Meditation and mindfulness are commonly recommended as a way of finding relief, both from the professionals and those who experience fatigue directly.

When I first started dabbling in mindfulness and meditation, they seemed like foreign concepts to my busy brain, but I soon learnt that these practices don't have to be difficult. The core focus is about being with yourself — still thinking, still dreaming, still planning your grocery list — just taking some valuable time out. You might say things like, '*I tried meditation*

---

48 This definition comes from the book, 'The Body Keeps the Score' by Bessel Van Der Kolk. If you can manage reading this book with your fatigue levels, it is one I highly recommend.
49 Definition based on the one provided in the Merriam-Webster dictionary, and true to my own experiences.

once and it wasn't for me' or even '*I failed*'. However, maybe it's simply about finding the right tool!

Over the years, I've found there are many methods of calming the mind and we just need to work out how. All of these methods have a direct effect on your nervous system, helping calm down any negative physiological responses that are adding to your fatigue levels.

I offer you the choice. There are multiple ways of being mindful and finding benefit in meditation. Here are nine ways of feeling mindful, each accompanied by a short introduction:

1. **Sitting mindfully** — *Sitting mindfully is all about relaxing, engaging your senses and being present in the moment.* Let's imagine you're sipping a hot drink. Notice the heat of the cup on your hands. Feel the warm liquid swirl inside your mouth. You might notice where you're sitting — the heat or cool of the air on your skin. You may hear noises– birds, the sound of traffic, a plane overhead, children laughing and playing. Noticing brings your attention to the here and now. It is a wonderful method for helping manage any anxious, ruminating thoughts.

2. **Guided meditation** — *Leading you with a spoken meditation experience.* Available online, there are many practitioners who offer guided services. I subscribe to a channel called 'The Mindful Movement' on YouTube.

3. **Yoga Nidra** — *A form of guided meditation that builds relaxation in your body.* You'll typically be lying down and completing a body scan, eventually slowing your mind's wavelengths to a sleep-like state. You can find guided yoga nidra tracks online.

4. **Moving mindfully** — *Using your body's movements to feel mindful and relaxed.* It may be dancing, or walking or any other type of movement that wakes up your body and feels good to you. Typically, you're present

in the moment, noticing what's around you and your own body's reactions.

5. **Technology** — *Using applications to assist and structure your mindfulness and mediation practice.* Common apps include Calm, Headspace and positive affirmation app ThinkUp.

6. **Mantras/chanting** — *Mantras and chanting[50] use words in your mind or out loud to calm the mind, body and soul.* You may have experienced the *Om* chant at the end of a yoga class and found the sound and vibration to be relaxing. Your mantra might be one word or a phrase that you adopt for yourself.

7. **Mindfulness meditation** — *Bringing your mind's attention to the present without drifting into concerns about the past or future.* This can be as simple as sitting or lying comfortably with your eyes closed, focusing on your breath and noticing how your body feels. This practice helps you break the train of everyday thoughts and helps you relax, using whatever technique feels right to you.

8. **Breathing techniques** — *Using patterns of breath to focus your mind inwards and physiologically change your body.* Breathing intentionally is a form of mindfulness and you can send energy around your body to help soften, ease and heal. An example might be to simply breathe in for 3, hold for 3 and out for 3, sending your breath to any areas of tension.

9. **Formal meditation practice** — *Dedicated to learning the skill and art of meditation.* If you want to formally learn meditation, there are any number of courses, books, retreats — great teachers to help you become the master of your own mind. This is where the benefits kick up a notch.

---

50 Brendan Burchard has a single word 'Release' meditation as an example of a mantra/chant — The link is here — https://www.youtube.com/watch?v=v2mY36Ho1Sk (Tip — Meditation starts at 10.50 in the video)

Many of these methods are easy for beginners to start with little or no experience behind them. If one option doesn't work, then just move onto another one. The trick is to find what works for you!

What ways of feeling mindful will you try?

As you can see above, there are multiple ways of achieving the same goal — bringing your attention back to the present moment and relaxing your mind and body.

Notice that a formal meditation practice only comes at the end. This is often the one you are told to start with, but there are many other easier practices to try that still bring great benefit.

Your goal is to enjoy trying out the different techniques, finding what works for you.

What works:

- **Find a practice that feels easy and restorative** — Try the nine ways above to see what works for you. The purpose is to find what helps bring you back into the present moment and relaxes your mind and body.
- **Carving out time each day for mindfulness and meditation** — Even if you only have five minutes a day, take that time to try out one of the techniques. You can work with activating triggers, such as first thing in the morning, when you have a hot drink in your hand, after a meal or just before you go to sleep.
- **Noticing your cues** — Anytime you notice tension, anxiety or when you are overwhelmed or stressed, you can take this as a cue to slow down and try one of these techniques.

What doesn't work:

- **Forcing meditation or mindfulness** — There are some days you might not feel mindful and that is okay. Forcing is never a good option and the opposite to what you want to achieve. I would suggest forgiving those days your mind is hectic, overworked or wont rest. Just try again the next day!

- **Expecting meditation to be emptying your mind** — Meditation is not about emptying your mind. All the time, people tell me they've tried it before, but their mind just doesn't sit still, so it's not for them. Good! You'd be dead! Instead of expecting nothingness, embrace the positive relaxation feelings it can bring you.

Chapter 20

Restoring Energy and Cultivating Joy

"I've now spent two years with long-COVID. I was initially supported by my wife of 21 years, but over the last year the cracks in our relationship that had been building for a while have led us to a permanent separation.

Separating is considered socially taboo in my culture, but in many ways, it was the best thing I could have done. This has been a healing pathway. While separating has not been easy, my headspace is so much better. I've found I have more peace, less anxiety as a result.

My wife and I have kept a healthy relationship, amicably navigating the separation for the sake of our two children who are now both in high school. Lately, my symptoms have been far less severe. I have more emotional energy to give both me and my children."

— Jin, 56, Japan

This topic is one that can be so sorely missed when dealing with long-term fatigue — connecting back in with what gives you energy, what makes you feel alive, what makes you thrive. In short, connecting with joy!

Dealing with long-term fatigue can mean we temporarily forget about the things that used to do this for us. Life can become focused on survival, more about navigating your condition than thriving.

Yes, it's difficult at times. Yes, it's even a long slog! Yes, it's all the challenges discussed so far. But life is also about your positive experiences and keeping your senses alive. Those sprinkles of joy that were mentioned in Chapter 15.

Finding your moments of energy and joy are an antidote to those darker days. It's always okay to feel negative emotions, but you don't need to live in this negative state. The question to ask yourself is, *'What do I need to do to shift myself out of this state into a more healing mindset?'*

This is a gentle reminder to make sure there is life in your day, even if you are confined to your house, on those days you feel most affected. Whatever you're feeling — despondent, fed up, in pain — there will be action you can take to bring you into a higher state of being, your healing mindset.

What transforms your mood on a rainy day?

What helps you transform your mood to this higher state will be as individual as you are. But let's start with five tried-and-true 'mood-lifters' that others and I have found useful.

Figure 26 — Five Mood-Lifters that Restore Energy and Cultivate Joy

1. **Music** — Whether it be actively listening to good beats, singing along or just enjoying a relaxing track in the background, music is a guaranteed way of changing your mood. The benefits include providing relaxation or distraction, lifting your spirits, even finding ways of processing complicated feelings. Music can also be a companion on the days when you feel most alone.

   Find the music that most 'speaks' to you and have your playlists on standby for the days you need it most.

2. **Laughter** — I like a big belly laugh every day and only need to look at the antics of my pups to find inspiration! Laughter releases the natural feel-good chemicals, helping you relax and dampen down stressful feelings.

   So many of us turn to humour as an effective way of coping with the marathon of peaks and troughs within long-term fatigue. This helps keep things in perspective and not 'waste' energy, our most precious commodity. It can even bring a sense of lightness to even the most challenging of situations.

   What do you have readily around you that amuses you? Is it watching a comedy show, listening to a light podcast, finding humour with loved ones, finding online videos, engaging in hobbies that make you laugh? Keeping your sense of humour alive is an essential tool in the management of any long-term condition.

3. **Gratitude** — It's difficult to feel simultaneously sad and grateful. Or frustrated and grateful. Or despairing and grateful… You get the picture.

   You might feel a confusing mix of emotions and it's okay to have strong negative feelings, such as grief or despair, about your current circumstances. You don't need to feel grateful for everything in life. Feeling grateful can start with the smallest of things — such as the softness of a comfortable bed, a friendly smile or a kind word, recognition of a nice sunny day, the taste of a good meal or the sound of birds chirping. Gratitude focuses you on the good in life — what is going right over what is going wrong. It eventually becomes a pattern of thinking that celebrates the good, helping you focus on what you want more of in your life.

4. **Creativity** — Here's something you might not have considered: finding ways to activate your creativity has a role to play in cultivating both energy and joy.

   You don't need to be a 'creative person' to do this either. Creativity comes in many different forms. It can be anything that sparks your imagination — writing or journaling, painting or other art forms, music, dance, exploring (in person or online), cooking, gardening, reading, problem-solving... The list goes on!

   Apart from being a distraction, when you're caught up in what you're doing, you can enter a deep state of flow, which is much like mindfulness. Find what sparks your creativity and imagination and build a bit of that into each day.

5. **Connection** — Connection with others provides emotional support and understanding. This is so useful for alleviating feelings of isolation. If you lack energy, it might mean that you fulfil your social needs in different ways. This may be about using the technology you have at your disposal, even if it's from your bed!

A couple of examples:

- Redefine how you spend Friday night 'drinks' with friends and use your phone or video call instead. Put your sparkling water in a fancy glass and away you go!
- Watch a movie or TV show with someone — even when not physically together, you can now stream shows at the same time.
- Engage in online forums to find others who face similar challenges. This can be such a relief and provide solid support.

You have the power to redefine how you build your supportive team — finding points of connection to ultimately build your energy and find joy.

Finding your favourite mood-lifters

These are all solid ways of lifting your state of being and building your healing mindset brick by brick. We've also discussed the other basic lifestyle factors that help with mood elevation, such as movement, nourishing foods, sleep, mindfulness, sunlight and getting out in nature.

Ultimately, the goal is finding ways of connecting with what makes you feel energised and joyful, bringing more of them into your day. Not all the mood-lifters discussed will necessarily work for you, and some are not tolerated with long-term fatigue either (think too much movement or ability to get out in the sun and nature).

You can start small and find what works for your situation. This may be your top two or three mood-lifters that are easy for you to start with, trying these daily or at least when you need to transform your mood.

What works

- **Find joy in small moments** — Sometimes it's the tiniest of things, our simplest pleasures that mean the most. It can be as small as an uplifting song, the feel of a hot drink, a sunrise/sunset, or reminding ourselves of a kind word from a friend.

- **Bringing yourself back to the present** — Focusing on the here and now (the sights, sounds, smells, textures) rather than ruminating on the past or future can restore a base of energy and joy. An easy way to do this is to close your eyes, focus on your breathing, taking a few deep mindful breaths to centre yourself. What can you hear? What can you feel? What can you smell? Think of one thing you love or are grateful for and sit with that for a while. When you open your eyes, you will feel more grounded, more mindful going forward.

- **Keeping stimulated and entertained** — Energy and joy can arise from finding what helps stimulate and entertain you. This can become about adapting what used to work to your new set of circumstances. Ideas for this include:

    - **Visual entertainment such as watching TV or reading** can be a great way of passing time when it's available to you. Just be aware of the cognitive load it carries. Where possible, keep it light rather than heavy on the drama and emotion, which we know can be draining. Comedy is a great genre for keeping your mood upbeat.

    - **Listening to podcasts or audio books** is a good option when you are extremely low in energy and want to keep your eyes closed, but also be entertained or learn something. This is fantastic for providing ambient noise that keeps you company without being taxing on your body. As with visual content, keep the topics light and easy to follow.

- **Prioritising self-care** — Set the foundation for energy and joy by focusing on the basic lifestyle factors that support your physical, mental, and emotional wellbeing (such as movement, nourishing food and good sleep). Finding what nurtures and rejuvenates you across these basics in turn helps you access your healing mindset.

What doesn't work

- **Pushing yourself to feel energised and joyful** — You're bound to have your negative moments, which honestly might be long moments! There's no need to try to force yourself to feel anything other than what you feel. Denying or ignoring your feelings often just makes them even worse. You can start small with your mood-lifters, and even just sleeping on a difficult day can mean you begin the next day with a fresh new perspective.

- **Comparison** — One of the unhelpful thought patterns, comparing your situation to others, or even to what you used to be able to do, is a one-way ticket to a negative state. The key is to redirect your focus using one of the mood-lifters to move past this state and feel better about your own progress and wellbeing.

Chapter 21
Maintaining Perspective

"I was diagnosed with ME/CFS in the final year of my architectural degree. It's been difficult watching my classmates enjoy an active social life and ace their exams while I'm stuck in a cycle of assignments, exams and constant crashes afterwards.

Lately, I've started to focus — eating a healthier diet, taking a range of supplements, and resting, resting, resting in my time off! This seems to be slowly paying off, and I'm feeling more energised over time. I now know how to better manage my energy. When I do inevitably crash, I also know how to handle it.

My last exam is next week, and after a long rest, I'll be taking up a local graduate position. While it's not been an easy journey, I'm feeling more grateful for this time that's taught me the importance of health and self-care. It's been a combination of patience and persistence that I never knew I had that's helped me get through."

— Thomas, 23, Denmark

We end how we began this book with a review of the marathon of improvement and personal recovery, discovering your new normal.

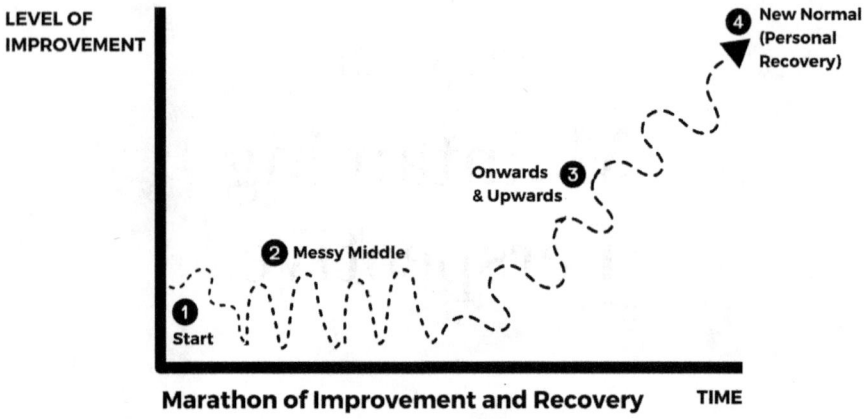

Figure 27 — Marathon of Improvement and Recovery

A quick overview of the four stages:

- **Stage 1** — Starting point…something is wrong
- **Stage 2** — Messy middle…peaks and troughs
- **Stage 3** — Onwards and upwards…consistent improvement over time
- **Stage 4** — New normal (personal recovery)…your new state of play

Stage 2 is the messy middle, but realistically your marathon journey has most likely been messy the whole way through. Progress is never a straight line, more like constant ups and downs, *'I'm fine, I'm not fine, I want to be fine so I will act fine (then collapse in a heap!).'*

If you look at the pattern of the typical journey in Figure 27, the improvement trend is not linear. It is indeed a twisted path full of peaks (improvements, celebration), but also troughs (regression, disappointment).

For many of us, there are periods of time where it seems like you are not getting any better. It may seem like two steps forward, one step back. Or even one step forward and two back! Your symptoms might even start worsening, or new symptoms start arising. You rebound or start feeling like there is improvement, only to find you crash again soon after.

Throughout this process, you are getting used to your limits. There are a new set of skills in energy management to learn. Pacing is now your new best friend! It may seem like there is constantly a learning curve, finding your invisible limits lest you pay the price of PEM revenge.

I outline this process to demonstrate from where it is that the emotional pain can arise. The crushing disappointment after you have a good day or even a good week, only to slip back into a dark period. The steps backward or the hitting the bottom of a dip on one of those messy middle curves.

To grieve is to be human, but these are also danger zones when it can be easy to lose perspective. And that's what's needed at every stage of your journey — **perspective.**

Smallest signs of improvement

One of the best ways to maintain your perspective is to recognise (and celebrate) even the smallest signs of improvement.

Improvements can be quite gradual and easy to miss, especially if you have been navigating your condition for quite some time. Perspective comes from actively recognising the good times as well as the bad.

Here are some examples of how these improvements might present:

- Doing an activity and not feeling PEM afterwards
- Being able to work on a task for 10 minutes

- Feeling bored with resting rather than absolutely needing the rest
- Feeling less tiredness after mental exertion, such as reading a book or working on your computer
- Being able to concentrate for longer periods of time
- Feeling greater mental clarity and ability to think clearly
- Feeling better able to focus on the people and conversations around you
- Reduction in pain and discomfort in your muscles and joints
- Improved stability of your mood, such as crying less or feeling more positive
- Increased motivation to engage in social events
- Improved sleeping patterns at night, such as being able to get to sleep and stay asleep
- Waking up in the morning feeling more refreshed
- Increased time doing physical activity and exercise with no (or minimal) PEM

What signs of improvement do you recognise?

You will notice that words like 'more', 'increased', 'greater' are used here as these improvements are all relative to your baseline of activity. You are **not** comparing these activities to what you used to be able to do and **definitely not** to what you would like to be able to do. Rather you are tracking your own progress over time, realistically considering the current stage of your condition.

It doesn't end at recognition either. You're also going to celebrate these smallest signs of improvement! If you wake up in the morning with slightly more pep in your step, that is a sign of improvement and worthy of celebration. If the next day you don't feel this pep, that's okay as well. As you probably know well by now, your daily experience can massively fluctuate. What you are looking for is that gradual improvement over time, particularly in Stage 3 onwards.

Recognising signs of improvement is an integral part of a healing mindset. It can become easy to lose yourself in the bad days, to focus on the negative experiences (of which I know there are most likely many). Your reality is filled with the light and shade of experiences and your perspective needs to reflect this. Learning to appreciate the improvements you feel on the upswing and not get thrown into the depths of despair on the downswing is a skill that will benefit you greatly through all that life throws at you.

It's a skill I've cultivated over time, but I'm not perfect at it. Even years on, I still get caught on occasion with tears and rumination over a period where I feel like I've regressed. The more improvement I feel, the harder it gets to have those low-energy days as I have so many things I want to do with my life. It's a marathon lesson indeed in perseverance and patience.

Your healing mindset holds perspective, but it's also a hopeful mindset, full of possibilities. It was a step I took towards feeling better about my condition — enjoying the good days and the improvements they brought. My experience is still not entirely without PEM or even dips in progress. Yet, rather than focusing on the negative, I celebrated in the extreme **any sign of improvement.** This included all those small milestones, such as waking up rested, being able to read a book in short bursts, attending a class at the gym and being able to spend a couple of hours with friends and family. Happy times indeed.

The role of trust in holding perspective

You can trust that you will have good days and bad days (or even a bad period), but you too will have an upward trajectory when your time is right. This notion of trust can be a hard one to come by. When you're in this messy middle, feeling the fatigue and all the other myriad of symptoms that accompany it, trusting that you will feel consistent improvement can be extremely difficult to do. This is true for anyone — you are not alone in this.

Trust at its core is about keeping your experience in perspective. It can be valuable to have someone close by to help you with this side of things. My partner Demian was incredible at pointing out my progress in my deepest moments of despair. Looking back, I can see how true that was — I was just in a trough and still trending upwards in improvement over time.

If you can, recruit someone to help you with this. If you don't have someone around, then not to worry — there are ways you can do this for yourself. Here are some tried-and-true methods of keeping this trust and perspective during your marathon event.

1. **Deputising someone to help you notice improvements** — This might involve explaining what improvement looks like for you and reviewing improvements with this person regularly. Ask them to point out how far you've come on your bad days.

2. **Keeping a diary of symptoms and severity and activity levels** — This helps with your medical appointments, but also reveals how you are tracking over time. It doesn't have to be onerous, rather a quick daily or weekly summary of how you are going. You can then track progress over the weeks, months or even over the year.

3. **Using technology to help** — Here are two applications that others have used to assist their fatigue journey.

    - **Visible** is an activity tracking platform for ME/CFS and long-COVID. Its core motto — *'Invisible illness. In plain sight.'* — reveals its aim, which is to make you and the people around you more aware of your experience. This application is still in beta at the time of writing.

- **Mind Pal** is a brain training game that challenges your memory, attention, language and problem-solving skills. It has been used to show evidence of progress, such as having less brain fog or increasing cognitive ability. Great for the more analytical among us who would like something concrete with which to measure progress.

Changing perspectives

What tends to happen over the marathon event is people tend to notice an upwards trajectory over time. In Stage 3 (onwards and upwards), the dips become less frequent, and the time taken to resolve these dips becomes shorter.

This is leading to your new normal, which usually involves a change in perspective. Your new normal requires reflection, even changing the fundamental way you view yourself — your self-image and identity.

Over time, your new normal allows you to re-engage with life, such as working, exercising and socialising more often. Your perspective will most likely have shifted and many changes in life become possible.

What's changing for you? Examples of such changes could include:

1. **Career changes** — Some people find they change focus. You may change the priority you put on work, or the hours you want to work. Maybe you want to change careers altogether, even make more (or less) of an impact on the world!
    - Changes in jobs and career
    - Changes in goals and dreams

2. **Lifestyle changes** — Some people experience a sea or tree change or downgrade their expectations around lifestyle. Going forward, the basics of good health you've been focusing on will stand you in good stead.

- Changes in lifestyle and views on health
- Changes in physical location
- Changes in support structures
- Changes in dependence on others
- Changes in financial circumstances

3. **Priority changes** — Your priorities may have changed. Often health becomes the top priority. Family and relationship bonds can also become your focus.

    - Changes in relationships
    - Changes in core focus
    - Changes in what is valued

4. **Knowledge level changes** — You're most likely now an expert at your own health. Pacing and resting are skills you apply naturally and subconsciously, and you've learnt how to create a sustainable pace in life.

    - Changes in what we see as our strengths
    - Changes in self-image and identity

Moving past asking 'when?'

Navigating these four stages, your marathon of peaks and troughs, can be a long and arduous experience with quite hazy timelines.

For me, not knowing these timelines has been one of my biggest challenges. In the first few years, I asked every medical professional that one question: when? *'When will I be fully recovered from this condition? When will my life go back to normal?'* No one has ever been able to give me an answer. It used to kill me every time.

If you're stuck on the asking 'when?' stage, I get it and I hope you can find peace with that question at some point soon. What you might find is your perspective changes over time to accept that life might never return to exactly how it was. You are moving and changing, and this itself opens you to new opportunities.

Your new normal will eventually come with a level of peace and acceptance — knowledge of how to nurture your tired body, focusing your valuable energy on the things that matter most and building a sustainable pace of life.

Eventually I started realising I didn't want my life to go back, and I had a new normal that was okay. I trained myself to stop asking that cursed question, instead just accepting. It took me a few years into my journey to come to these resolutions, but this acceptance provided me valuable peace of mind and the opportunity to craft a different, more sustainable focus in life.

What works

- **Writing down your signs of improvement** — Easy to miss, signs of improvement are everywhere and are important to recognise and celebrate. A good practice is to write down even the smallest of improvements — waking up feeling slightly energised, being able to make a hot drink and sit with it quietly, an outing you were able to attend. All of these become important milestones and a cause for celebration.

- **Deputising someone to help you hold perspective** — An outside point of view will hold more perspective in the times you feel down, even if it's your own words in your journal. If it's another person, show them the marathon journey in Figure 27 and get them to explain back to you that you are just in a trough during the times when you feel like you are losing your perspective.

- **Reaching the goal of acceptance** — There is a certain peace with accepting what is and what will be rather than wishing for something different. The ultimate goal is to accept this is your journey for now, holding trust that things will not always be this way.

- **Embracing changing perspectives** — The gift of acceptance is that it often is the catalyst to new opportunities. Your new normal often comes with a whole suite of changes, including career, lifestyle, priority and knowledge level changes. Embracing these changes takes time and might not seem possible right now. But hold hope for the possibilities that can arise once you are ready for your new normal.

What doesn't work

- **Maintaining a negative outlook** — Long-term conditions are challenging to our sense of self-image and identity. You might reflect and realise the strength and resilience shown navigating such a marathon event. Or it may be that you are stuck feeling weak and vulnerable from the same circumstances. Both views are possible, but only one will give you the energy you need to make the most of your current circumstances. Focusing on the negative becomes disempowering and adds to fatigue over time.

- **Getting caught on the 'when?'** — While understandable, focusing on when you will be fully recovered is usually a futile action as no one can reliably answer that question. A better focus becomes living in the moment, recognising and enjoying those small signs of improvement that you can see along the way.

New Reality — A Message of Hope

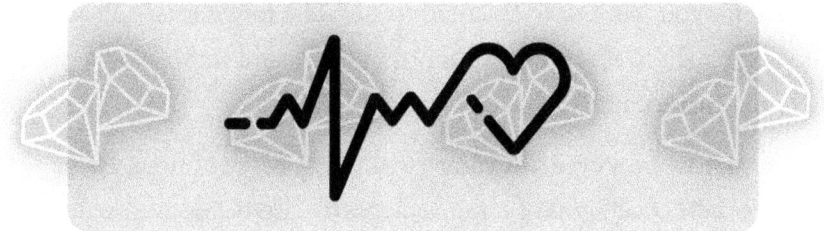

As my energy comes back, at first sporadically and now more steadily, I dip my toe tentatively into the stream of life that flows around me. I'm starting to trust again — trust my energy, trust my abilities, trust my purpose.

And I'm not alone! Stories are mounting of people who have reached their new normal — maybe not quite how they were previously, but a new flow of life. No longer too tired to think.

It's okay if this is not you right now. Long-term management of any condition is difficult and everyone with fatigue goes through their own journey on their own timeline. In particular, the messy middle part of your marathon journey takes time. If any professional gives you a timeframe for your recovery, they are doing you a disservice, as the 'when' of recovery is difficult to predict.

Evidence demonstrates that people do emerge from fatigue feeling substantial improvement. For some, that means full recovery. For others, we've defined our own new normal, knowing we can still lead happy and productive lives. All of us who have done so are living, breathing examples of what is possible with time. Knowing this hopefully provides you with some level of comfort. I can only urge you to never, never give up — there is always a reason to look forward.

We are each on a sliding scale of wellness — it's never absolute. You'll have good days and bad. Your healing mindset allows you to own how bad you truly feel, but not dwell there indefinitely. To try treatments recommended for you, but not to be afraid to advocate for yourself and stop if it's not working. To live each day around your limits and embrace what you can do, rather than ruminating over what you cannot.

Ultimately, improvement comes with the passage of time. It's your job to notice these small signs of improvement. It's also being consistent in your lifestyle choices, trying new ways of treating your condition and holding on to hope even during those times when you feel your weakest.

It starts with just one moment, one hour, one day at a time. A unicorn day emerges when your energy picks up and you get something done. Hallelujah! You marvel at your achievement with pure joy as it's the simple things in life that now mean the most. You make a tasty meal, see a friend, get out into the sunshine, drink a cappuccino, play some music, even dance a bit. You don't know what tomorrow will hold, but you are eternally grateful for today.

Once your energy emerges, even just a little, the things you can do! The first time you can attend an event and feel halfway decent the next day. You resume an activity knowing you will be able to commit to it. Or even realising that you've had a busy day and now feel tired, but not 'chronic fatigue' tired.

Maybe you're cautious at first, not quite trusting (and nor should you). You're tentative, hesitant, full of fear and angst. Gradually, you start to believe in your energy again, in your body, but mostly in your ability to handle the odd crash.

You become willing to push your limits just to see what's possible. Sometimes you're pleasantly surprised and other times you overdo it, feeling the effects. This becomes no big deal. It was too much and you won't do that again in a hurry!

Over time, you become more willing to trust — what a heady feeling of joyous elation that becomes! Eventually, finding those limits becomes subconscious and effortless. You're unleashed!

Timing is everything. If you'd suggested I write this book at the peak of my chronic fatigue journey, you might as well have told me to get into my spaceship and fly to Jupiter! It's taken seven years of time and a whole load of patience I didn't want to have. This is where trust in the 'when' becomes a leap of faith, year after year trusting that a level of recovery will eventuate when the time is right.

I'm still affected today and even endure the odd crash — gaining more lessons around my limits. It can seem like I'm thrown back into the marathon when I have a string of bad days in a row, becoming all too easy to lose sight of the bigger picture and focus just on the painful weakness in my body. It's a test that I've learnt how to pass — falling back on my lifestyle basics, my healing mindset, my expert pacing skills and (patiently?) waiting for the next day to bring me back to life.

"No pressure, no diamonds," philosopher Thomas Carlyle once said. My time with long-term fatigue and beyond has most definitely been a diamond in the making. As I look back at the magic and hell of that time, it helps me recognise my progress, the lessons I was forced into learning! Lately, I feel like a flower unfurling in the sun. I'm in love with my body and all its capabilities. I no longer resent the weakness it holds. Resentment, hate, bad feelings are done and I'm moving into the light!

As I sit here writing this, energy powers through my veins. I feel powerful with intent — my message is needed in this world, and I must deliver it! The last few years have fundamentally changed my outlook on life. I waste my energy no more — it's the ultimate resource after all. I feel flow and love and excited for a future that picks up travel and adventure again. I'm more aware of my physical body and those pesky limits. I don't take being able to do anything for granted and this allows me to look at the world with greater awe and gratitude.

How you look back on your time with fatigue will vary. For some, it's a blip; for others, it's a transforming experience. It might even be a time of life that leads to new meaning — our sixth stage of the grief cycle.

Ultimately, the lens through which you view your time with your condition will change, even soften. There are lessons learnt that we take through to the next life chapter, whatever that holds. These are gifts — ones you didn't ask for maybe but receive nonetheless.

These gifts come in the form of new skills developed, different relationships, more mindfulness and self-compassion. There's the ability to recognise and celebrate small successes, less hustle and a slower pace of life, more downtime. It's listening to what your body needs and delivering on it, unflinchingly prioritising your health and wellbeing, and never never taking your health or energy for granted. In short, conscious living that leads to more joy.

Lessons you take forward will define your next chapter. You're aiming for acceptance, but allow yourself to ride the rollercoaster of emotions. You're no doubt aware that mindset training is an ongoing project; you will most likely find there is always more work to do. Remember to look for that insidious unhelpful programming and train your mind to make a different choice — a gentler, more healing way of thinking. Sounds easy for something that takes a lifetime of practice!

This is our new reality — people rising from their beds, leaving their wheelchairs behind, feeling ready to take on the world again and creating their new normal. You might emerge changed, but are you ever the same person you were ten or even five years ago? No, you have always been constantly evolving. You will have endured, become stronger, more definite in what you need and are willing to give. Your body will tell you when it's time. Your job is to listen and believe in what's possible.

It is then that the whole world awaits.

Acknowledgments

I didn't set out to write this book, but somehow it started flowing through me and it became my job to be a conduit for this message. I have followed this course faithfully, knowing there are people who will benefit from my experience.

But it hasn't been all flow! The burden of creating a book has been a *huge* learning curve, both exhilarating and uncomfortable at the same time.

You never do these things alone and I've been gifted invaluable help with the content. I would firstly like to recognise the (devastatingly honest) stories from those experiencing long-term fatigue shared with me personally or via Facebook groups. Over the years, interviewing individuals and being in the groups have allowed me to not only feel seen, but also supplement my own stories and incorporate the research of hundreds (if not thousands) of situations into the content.

While crafting the structure and content, I want to recognise the following people who have been part of the process from beta readers, to proofreading, to content review: Rachel Collard, Caitlin Bauer, Neil James, Brad Kerwin, Deborah Daly, Sabino Garcia, Erika Bass, Judith Stevens, and Terri Tonkin. A massive thank you. This book has a much stronger narrative through your input.

To Mark Clisby from Emerge who was an advance reader and a great source of advice and wisdom, thank you. I value the ongoing advocacy that

Emerge provides. If you have a long-term fatigue condition, please consider becoming a member of Emerge for the support they can provide.

To my amazing editor, Kris Emery Editorial. Kris has been so patient with the process, helped smooth those rough edges and create the easy-to-read and helpful guide you see today.

Thank you also to my incredible sister-in-law Helen Vizer and her impressive attention-to-detail as a proofreader. Helen has been a great support over the last few years. In times of my greatest fatigue, her weekly calls helped keep a sense of connection. Speaking of family, a shout out to my brother John who just wanted to see his name in print, somewhere, sometime!

A big thank you to Tracey Spicer for the initial push. The fact Tracey was so willing to share her long-COVID journey, warts and all, inspired me to be equally vulnerable and brave. Before Tracey's story, my dominant feeling was shame for what has been such a difficult time of life.

To my partner Demian Coorey, always so supportive on the home front and who continues to believe I'm the most energetic person in the room! My beautiful pup Oliver Queen was my constant companion in those earlier difficult years, and I'd hate to think where I'd be without him. We are joined by our latest pup Savannah who has been of little help, mostly full of naughtiness. Lucky she's cute! These three are my family, my life.

Thank you to all my friends and family who continue to ask how the book is going. 'It's a slow process' was my standard reply, but clearly now I've reached the finish line!

Finally, thank *you* for choosing to read this book. Writing this has given me a sense of purpose, a reason to record my experiences. It's kept me going at times. For this, I am truly grateful. My aim is to provide you a sense of hope in return for reading, but I also wanted to adequately reflect your reality, however that looks for you. My message remains this...

Keep going, no matter what, knowing you are not alone.

Sarah Vizer, November 2024

Glossary

Acceptance and commitment therapy (ACT) — A type of mindful psychotherapy that uses mindfulness exercises to help you process difficult emotions by staying focused in the present, accepting thoughts and feelings without judgements. Like CBT, it can be used by people with long-term fatigue to help adjust and cope with their condition, but is not considered a treatment or cure for the underlying condition.

Baseline level of energy — The amount of energy you have at any one point in time for daily activity. This is most likely a mix of activities such as self-care, working, household chores, responsibilities relating to looking after children/pets and social occasions. This may be a lot lower with long-term fatigue than what you are used to have previously.

Boom-and-bust — The cycle that develops when you expend large amounts of energy over a short period of time (boom), followed by necessary rest or inactivity to recover (bust). A perpetual cycle of boom-and-bust occurs when you are constantly pushing yourself to get through the day, then crashing and recovering just enough, but never actually feeling like you're fully restoring enough energy to stop the cycle.

Cognitive behavioural therapy (CBT) — A common type of talk-therapy or psychotherapy that looks to help change unhelpful or unhealthy ways of thinking, feeling and behaving. CBT can be an effective tool to help treat mental health conditions, such as PTSD, depression or anxiety. It can support you to adjust and cope with your condition, but it not considered a treatment or cure for fatigue conditions in itself.

Cognitive distortion — Creating a negative or pessimistic filter that distorts your current reality. Unhelpful thinking patterns contribute to creating distortion in how you view your fatigue condition.

Conventional/Western/Allopathic medicine — Science-based medicine that is practiced by professionals who have obtained a medical degree from a recognised medical school and are licensed to practice in their respective countries. Your primary care doctor will typically practice this type of medicine.

Crash — The feeling of complete exhaustion that occurs when you exhaust your energy envelope (the amount of energy you have available) and have no choice but to rest as a result. At its worst, this can last for several days or even weeks for an intense recovery period.

Dark days — The inevitable days when life's circumstances can feel difficult to manage. They may promote those unhelpful and unsupportive thinking patterns.

Deconditioning — Decline in physical function of the body as a result of physical inactivity and/or bedrest or an extremely sedentary lifestyle.

Emotion-focused therapy (EFT) — A type of therapy focused on making sense of your emotions and their role in your human experience and change. Like CBT and ACT, it is sought out by some people with long-term fatigue to help adjust and cope with their condition, but is not considered a treatment or cure for the underlying condition.

Energy envelope — The amount of energy you have available each day. When you have a fatigue condition, your energy envelope will likely be substantially lower than what it used to be.

Fibromyalgia — A disorder of the central nervous system characterised by chronic widespread musculoskeletal pain and joint swelling. It is commonly accompanied by fatigue and can also coexist with a whole range of other issues.

Functional medicine — A science-based medicine that takes a holistic approach, integrating conventional medicine with alternate and complementary therapies.

Gems — Practitioners who are dedicated to helping their patients and will show kindness and compassion for your condition. They can recognise fatigue is a complex condition, can help you with an accurate diagnosis and will provide suggestions on how to treat your fatigue.

Golden rule of energy — My energy rule for people and situations; to only do things or have interactions which give you more energy than they require from you.

Graded exercise therapy (GET) — Physical therapy that aims to increase your stamina and prevent or reverse deconditioning and exercise intolerance. It involves setting a baseline of activity, which is improved upon over time. GET is increasingly not recommended as a treatment for those with long-term fatigue conditions as it can lead to distress and even harm when it is results to PEM. Pacing and rest are recommended instead.

Grief cycle — A model developed by the Swiss-American psychiatrist Elizabeth Kübler-Ross around the cycle of human emotional states, or the five stages of grief. The stages have application beyond grief, including capturing the mix of emotions when navigating big life changes such as fatigue. You will jump back and forth between the five stages, those being denial, anger, bargaining, depression and acceptance. A sixth stage, meaning, has also been proposed.

Healing mindset — A way of thinking that promotes healing, growth and wellbeing. It involves focusing on helpful, constructive thoughts and actions, rather than negative or unhelpful thought patterns.

Improvement — In relation to your fatigue condition, a substantial reduction in baseline symptoms, along with partial restoration of everyday activities, with or without pacing or medication.

Integrative medicine — A type of medicine with conventionally trained medical practitioners who have completed more training and are therefore considered more of a specialist. They combine treatments from conventional medicine with alternative or complementary therapies where there is high-quality evidence of safety and effectiveness.

Long-term fatigue — Extreme fatigue lasting longer than six months, with symptoms that worsen through physical or mental activity and that are not relieved by rest or sleep.

Meditation — The practice of connecting with, being with and recharging yourself. It uses a combination of mental and physical techniques (such as concentrating on your breathing or repetition of a mantra) for the purpose of reaching a heightened level of spiritual awareness.

Mindfulness — A quality of paying attention in a moment. It involves being able to hover calmly and objectively over your thoughts, feelings and emotions.

Mindset — Also known as your frame of mind, is the perceptions and beliefs that shape how you make sense of the world and yourself. This creates a way of thinking around your fatigue condition. Your mindset is never all good or all bad and can be a mix of both positive and negative, sometimes even simultaneously.

Misdiagnosis — The state of play where your fatigue condition is not recognised, or your symptoms attributed to an incorrect cause, such as psychological rather than physical issues. It can also be a failure to recognise the severity of your condition, such as 'trouble sleeping' rather than a more realistic 'extreme and unrelenting fatigue'.

Myalgic encephalomyelitis/chronic fatigue syndrome (ME/CFS) — A complex medical condition characterised by severe, persistent fatigue, with symptoms that worsen with physical and mental activity and don't fully improve with rest.

Multidisciplinary approach — Occurs when you utilise a range of different practitioners to find medical and emotional support and make needed lifestyle changes. The goal is to use the full spectrum of options available to treat the symptoms and help improve your overall quality of life.

New normal — Reaching a point of improvement that might not feel like full recovery in the truest sense. In your new normal, you still live with symptoms of fatigue, but have transformed your outlook on what life entails compared to before your condition. You are effectively embracing a new reality, adapting life around the limitations of your condition.

Long-COVID — A condition arising from SARS-CoV-2 (COVID-19) infections. It is a continuation or development of new symptoms three months after the initial COVID-19 infection. It is commonly accompanied by fatigue and can also coexist with a wide range of other symptoms.

Pacing — A self-management strategy that establishes a routine of activity to balance activity and rest, matching your current energy levels.

Post-exertional malaise (PEM) — The after-effects of physical, mental or emotional exertion. These effects can last for hours, days or even weeks at a time.

Postural orthostatic tachycardia syndrome (POTS) — A serious medical condition whereby your heart races, you feel dizzy or weak, you might shake or sweat with even the slightest of exertion. It can be triggered by as little as walking up a set of stairs and other factors such as dehydration, prolonged bed rest and certain medications.

Practitioners — An umbrella term, used to describe all the different professionals, medical or otherwise, that form part of your treatment team. Examples include your primary care doctor, dietitians, health coaches, yoga teachers, exercise physiologists and psychologists.

Primary care doctor — Usually a conventionally trained doctor that becomes your central point of contact for all things medically related. They can coordinate with other practitioners and make sure anything you try is safe and appropriate for your condition.

Productive conversations — Conversations with either yourself or someone else that become more analytical and work through your experience rather than pure venting. Outcomes of productive conversations include creating greater understanding, being able to better process your emotions and being able to employ the strategy of reframing.

Recovery — In relation to your fatigue condition, full recovery means not experiencing PEM for six months and being able to perform what used to be your normal levels of activity without pacing or medication.

Reframing — Looking at an issue or event in a new way or from another angle in order to find a different perspective. A healing mindset is often about reframing to find the angle that looks through a gentler, more generous or positive lens.

Rocks — Practitioners who at best have not been able to help you. At worst, they weigh you down, even actively set you back in some way, such as being dismissive or uneducated around long-term fatigue.

Self-sabotage — The unhelpful programming that creeps into your mind, creating negative thought patterns or a negative mindset around your situation. This can result in negative emotions such as guilt or frustration as well as judgements around your condition, particularly around what you can no longer do.

TATT — An acronym for 'tired all the time', which is a common and non-specific symptom that is presented to medical practitioners by their patients.

Traditional medicines (also known as natural medicine) — Medical practices that typically work alongside conventional medicine to complement the approach, or in the case of alternative medicine offer a different solution. Examples include alternative medicine (e.g. traditional Chinese medicine), complementary medicine and naturopathic medicine.

Unhelpful thought patterns — Ways your thoughts become biased and form a negative mindset around your fatigue condition. Examples include believing things 'should' be a certain way, exaggerating the negative aspects and catastrophising situations, or personalising by feeling responsible for what's not your fault or within your control.

About the author

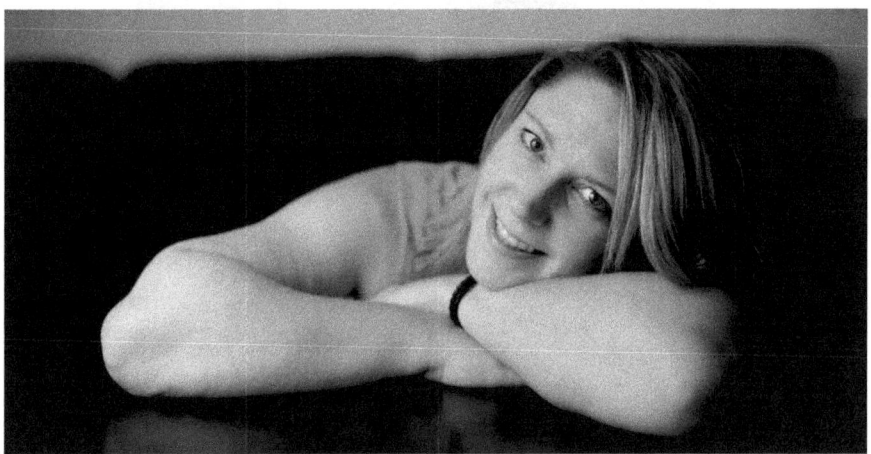

Sarah Vizer is an author, executive coach and consultant.

Too Tired to Think has stemmed from Sarah's story of corporate burnout, which led to her on-going battle with chronic fatigue syndrome. She is intimately familiar with the challenges fatigue presents and now shares her story to inspire others to improve their wellbeing and build a brighter future.

Sarah is a well-regarded thought leader on the topics of burnout and long-term fatigue. She draws on her expertise in mindset, health psychology, and behavioural change to create comprehensive solutions that untangle complexity and captures the human side of her subjects. She has a knack for being able to resonate with her readers on a deeply personal level.

Sarah lives and writes out of Brisbane, Australia with her partner and fur children. You can visit her at: www.sarahvizer.com

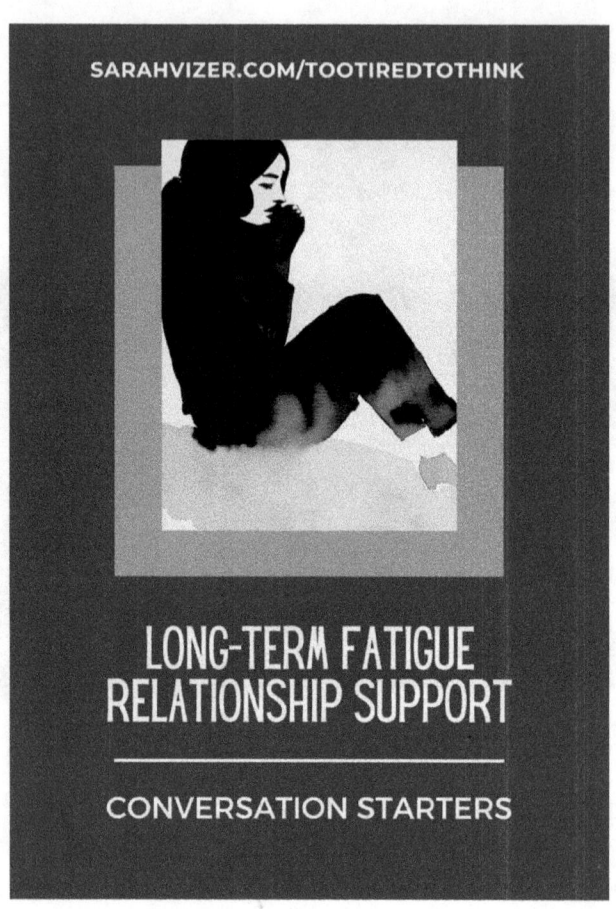

Free downloadable e-book

A bonus e-book provides scripts and conversations starters that will spark valuable discussions with the important people in your life.

This insightful resource will help create shared understanding, deeper bonds and mutual support.

You can get your copy at: www.sarahvizer.com/tootiredtothink

www.ingramcontent.com/pod-product-compliance
Lightning Source LLC
Chambersburg PA
CBHW070759040426
42333CB00060B/961